HEALTHCARE
STRATEGIC
PLANNING

HEALTHCARE
STRATEGIC
PLANNING

FOURTH EDITION

JOHN M. HARRIS, Editor

Contributing Authors
Katherine A. Cwiek
Carol N. Davis
Mark J. Dubow
Scott Stuecher

ACHE Management Series

The paper used in this publication meets the minimum requirements of American National Standard for Information Sciences—Permanence of Paper for Printed Library Materials, ANSI Z39.48-1984. ∞ ™

Acquisitions editor: Janet Davis; Project manager: Theresa L. Rothschadl; Cover designer: James Slate; Layout: PerfecType

Found an error or a typo? We want to know! Please e-mail it to hapbooks@ache.org, mentioning the book's title and putting "Book Error" in the subject line.

For photocopying and copyright information, please contact Copyright Clearance Center at www.copyright.com or at (978) 750–8400.

Health Administration Press
A division of the Foundation of the American
   College of Healthcare Executives
300 S. Riverside Plaza, Suite 1900
Chicago, IL 60606–6698
(312) 424–2800

Contents

Section 4   Optimizing Strategic Planning

Preface

Earlier editions of *Healthcare Strategic Planning* are dog-eared and underlined in the offices of many healthcare CEOs and strategic planners. As healthcare leaders wrestle with rapid and profound changes, they must help their organizations develop and implement effective strategies to thrive. This fourth edition provides a how-to guide for healthcare organizations seeking to undertake strategic planning in our dynamic environment.

In this revision, we provide core insights into strategic planning practice and theory and into how those insights can be applied to healthcare organizations. In addition to a step-by-step presentation of the planning process, the book includes essential advice on critical aspects of successful planning, such as stimulating truly strategic thinking, executing implementation, transitioning to strategic management, and maximizing results through annual plan updates.

We have also updated this edition to address contemporary issues, including population health, value-based payment, and provider–payer partnerships. An entire chapter is devoted to innovations in healthcare business models and technologies. The latest research on healthcare strategic planning is punctuated with contemporary examples from our experience assisting Veralon clients. These examples provide fresh insights into how healthcare organizations are conducting strategic planning and using their strategies to leapfrog into the future, staying ahead of competitors.

The tools in the new edition will help CEOs, planners, physicians, trustees, and other professionals understand key concepts and make the planning process a robust learning and growth experience for their organizations.

In the five years since the previous edition, our views on the strategic planning process have evolved, based on the insights of Veralon consultants who apply the process, as well as on feedback from the clients with whom the process was used. This edition of the book reflects that evolution.

First, to make this edition easier to navigate, we have grouped the chapters into the following four major sections:

- Section 1—Making the Case for Strategic Planning
  In addition to helping the reader understand the benefits of strategic planning, this section can help convince organizational leaders to invest sufficient time and resources to get the full benefit of an effective planning process.

- Section 2—Setting the Stage for Successful Strategic Planning
  Preparation is vital to successful planning. This section describes the key decisions and preparation required for a successful process and plan.

- Section 3—The Strategic Planning Process
  The four phases of strategic planning—analyzing the environment, setting organizational direction, formulating strategy, and implementation—are described in clear steps with real-life examples from our work with clients.

- Section 4—Optimizing Strategic Planning
  For more advanced planners, this section addresses topics that can help an organization get even more out of strategic planning.

We have refined and added helpful content in every chapter, with approximately 30 pages of additional content. Key changes include:

- Chapter 1—The Value of Strategic Planning

  This chapter has been renamed to reflect our increased emphasis on the value and benefits of strategic planning. We have also addressed why and how healthcare strategic planning is different from strategic planning in other industries, based on new research.

- Chapter 2—Benefits of Strategic Planning

  In this chapter, we have included new graphics illustrating new concepts, case studies illustrating more contemporary situations with an emphasis on population health management, and clear summaries of the benefits of strategic planning.

- Chapter 3—Organizing for Success

  We have reorganized the 12 steps involved in preparing for strategic planning under four categories, simplifying planning execution.

- Chapter 4—Major Planning Process Considerations

  We have updated examples, tools, and research, with a new focus on stakeholders.

- Chapter 5—Encouraging Strategic Thinking

  We have provided new research on incorporating truly strategic thinking into planning and ongoing management.

- Chapter 6—Phase 1: Analyzing the Environment

  We have provided updated examples, including new exhibits of strategic frameworks, and expanded the approach to quantitative analysis in this chapter.

- Chapter 7—Phase 2: Organizational Direction
  We have updated and added examples and restructured the chapter for a smoother read.

- Chapter 8—Phase 3: Strategy Formulation
  This entire chapter was updated with new examples and real-world case studies that incorporate current strategic issues and provide a detailed picture that helps readers envision key strategic plan outputs.

- Chapter 9—Phase 4: Transition to Implementation
  We have recognized successful implementation as one of the greatest challenges for organizations completing strategic plans. Based on our client experiences, we added a step-by-step process for developing effective implementation plans.

- Chapter 10—Annual Review and Update
  Based on lessons learned in the field, we have added new ideas for integrating implementation plans into other organizational work processes to ensure that strategic plans are actually implemented.

- Chapter 11—Enabling More Effective Execution
  We have included lessons from outside the healthcare field on keeping the strategic plan up-to-date. We have also included new case studies with a key example of one highly developed system's annual strategic planning process.

- Chapter 12—Addressing Innovation in Strategic Planning
  This new chapter discusses game-changing innovations that will create new winners and losers in the healthcare sector. Two types of innovation are explored: business model innovation, particularly related to alignment of

providers and payers, and clinical and technological innovations that may change healthcare.

- Chapter 13—Future Challenges for Strategic Planners
  We have summarized and elaborated on new research and recommendations for the future for healthcare strategic planners and strategists, including special skills required.

We hope you enjoy the fourth edition of *Healthcare Strategic Planning*. Five years of interaction with clients, presentation audiences, and colleagues have offered much grist for the mill in updating this book.

Special thanks are due to the many consultants of Veralon who expand our insights and techniques for successful strategic planning in every client engagement. I particularly want to thank those members of the Veralon team who are contributing authors for this edition: Scott Stuecher, manager; Mark Dubow, director; Carol Davis, principal; and Katherine Cwiek, former manager. In addition, Dana Rosenbaum provided extensive organizational and research support for this edition.

We thank those clients that have allowed us to write about their real-life experiences and insights so that others may learn. We particularly acknowledge:

Ascension
Hunterdon Healthcare System
Jefferson Health
McDonough District Hospital
St. Mary's Health System (Evansville, Indiana)
Stony Brook Medicine
UW Health
Yavapai Regional Medical Center

Finally, we express our sincere gratitude to all clients of Veralon. By responding to your questions and needs, we customize and refine our approaches, gaining insights that we have the privilege of sharing through this book.

John M. Harris
Philadelphia, Pennsylvania

Making the Case for Strategic Planning

CHAPTER 1

The Value of Strategic Planning

The organization without a strategy is willing to try anything.

—Michael Porter

*There is surely nothing quite so useless as doing with
great efficiency that which should not be done at all.*

—Peter Drucker

For decades, top scholars and strategy experts have debated the bottom line value of strategic planning and whether planning is an effective way to craft good strategy. Understanding concerns raised about the efficacy of strategic planning (notably Martin 2014; Mintzberg 1994) can be useful because, although criticisms do not invalidate strategic planning as a path to sound strategy, they do call attention to what can make planning fail. Thus, criticisms highlight how planning must be designed and executed to overcome potential pitfalls on the journey to meaningful strategy, and they can also heighten awareness of challenges in a way that is beneficial to students of strategy and planners alike.

Before one is able to appreciate why strategic planning is in fact a viable path to good strategy, however, establishing a common understanding of the more foundational elements is important—what strategy is, what defines *good* strategy, and what strategic planning is.

WHAT IS STRATEGY?

Though this book primarily focuses on the *process* rather than the *content* of strategy (as distinguished by Mintzberg 1978, 1994; Mintzberg, Ahlstrand, and Lampel 1998; Porter 1979, 1998), and specifically on the strategic planning process for healthcare organizations, defining the latter is critical to evaluating the value of the former.

The concept of strategy has roots primarily in military history and secondarily in political history. "The English word strategy comes from the Greek *strategos*, meaning a general . . . and the Greek verb *strategeo* means to plan the destruction of one's enemies through effective use of resources. Many terms used in strategy today—objectives, mission, strengths, weaknesses—also have military roots" (Ginter, Duncan, and Swayne 2013, 7).

For purposes of business, Wickham Skinner (1969, 140) defined strategy as a "set of plans and policies by which a company aims to gain advantages over its competitors." Porter (1996, 70) asserts that "the essence of strategy is choosing what not to do" and that strategy is about making the choices necessary to distinguish an organization in meeting customers' needs. Others describe strategy more pragmatically as answering questions of where we are going and how we get there (Eisenhardt 1999). The defining attribute of strategy—the "nucleus" (Porter 1996) or "kernel" (Rumelt 2011a)—relates to establishing and leveraging sustainable competitive advantage and fulfilling the intention of a firm's strategic direction (Hamel and Prahalad 1989).

WHAT IS GOOD STRATEGY?

The authors of this book, adapting the framework proffered by J. Daniel Beckham (2000), propose seven key characteristics of effective strategy:

1. *Sustainability.* It has lasting power with greater long-term impact than other alternatives.
2. *Performance benefits.* It yields improvement on key performance and competitive position indicators.
3. *Competitive advantages.* Its approach is demonstrably unique and superior to those employed by competitors and thus yields competitive advantages.
4. *Direction.* It moves the organization toward a defined end, although not necessarily in a linear fashion.
5. *Focus.* It is targeted and represents a choice to pursue a certain course over other attractive alternatives.
6. *Interconnectedness.* Its components have a high level of interdependence and synergy.
7. *Criticality.* It may not be essential to organizational success, but it is certainly significant and fundamental.

In *Good Strategy, Bad Strategy*, Richard Rumelt (2011a) asserts that good strategy has a sound underlying logic and structure that make up the "kernel" of a strategy. A good strategy may consist of more than the kernel, but if the kernel is absent or misshapen, problems will ensue. The kernel of a strategy contains three elements: (1) a diagnosis that defines or explains the nature of the challenge, (2) a guiding policy for dealing with the challenge, and (3) a set of coherent actions that are designed to carry out the guiding policy.

Rumelt (2011b, 5) further elaborates, "A good strategy does more than urge us forward toward a goal or vision. A good strategy honestly acknowledges the challenges being faced and provides an approach to overcoming them. And the greater the challenge, the more a good strategy focuses and coordinates efforts to achieve a powerful competitive punch or problem-solving effect."

WHAT IS STRATEGIC PLANNING?

A number of definitions have evolved to pinpoint the essence of strategic planning. According to Peter M. Ginter, W. Jack Duncan, and Linda E. Swayne (2013, 21), "Strategic planning defines where the organization is going, sometimes where it is not going, and provides focus. The plan sets direction for the organization and—through a common understanding of the vision and broad strategic goals—provides a template for everyone in the organization to make consistent decisions that move the organization toward its envisioned future. Strategic planning, in large part, is a decision-making activity."

Beckham (2016) describes true strategy as "a plan for getting from a point in the present to some point in the future in the face of uncertainty and resistance." A. B. Campbell (1993) adds the concept of measurement to his definition, which characterizes strategic planning as a process for defining an organization's objectives, the strategies to achieve objectives, and metrics that gauge effectiveness of strategies.

Connie Evashwick and W. T. Evashwick (1988), incorporating the concepts of vision and mission, propose that strategic planning creates a vision of the future based on how the organization fits into its current and anticipated environment given its mission, strengths, and weaknesses. Once a vision is in place, the organization develops a plan of action to position itself accordingly.

Many variations of the strategic planning model exist and are used, but all have common core tenets. Two similar approaches to strategic planning were developed in the 1980s. The first, proposed by Donna L. Sorkin, Nancy Ferris, and James Hudak (1984), features the following steps:

- Scan the environment.
- Undertake external and internal analyses.
- Select key issues.
- Set a mission statement and broad goals.
- Develop goals, objectives, and strategies for each issue.
- Develop an implementation plan to carry out strategic actions.
- Monitor, update, and scan.

The second approach was tailored to healthcare and included these steps (Simyar, Lloyd-Jones, and Caro 1988):

- Identify the organization's current position, including present mission, long-term objectives, strategies, and policies.
- Analyze the environment.
- Conduct an organizational audit.
- Identify the various alternative strategies based on relevant data.
- Select the best alternative.
- Gain acceptance.
- Prepare long-range and short-range plans to support and carry out the strategy.
- Implement the plan and conduct an ongoing evaluation.

This book synthesizes steps from the two approaches into four stages, as illustrated in exhibit 1.1.

The first stage is the environmental assessment, which focuses on the question, where are we now? It has three primary outputs:

1. Evaluation of competitive position, including advantages and disadvantages
2. Assumptions about the future environment
3. Distillation of key strategic issues to address

The goal of the environmental assessment is to determine how an organization may fare in the future given likely conditions and current position and to pinpoint the factors most critical to generating future competitive advantage.

The second stage of the planning process is organizational direction, followed by the third stage, strategy formulation. Stages 2 and 3 address the question, where should we be going? The main activity of the organizational direction stage is to define a desired future state by examining possible future external realities, mission,

Exhibit 1.1: The Strategic Planning Approach

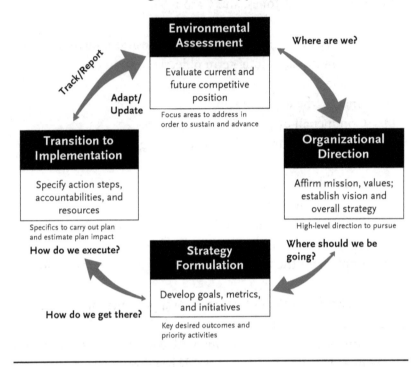

Environmental Assessment — Evaluate current and future competitive position — Focus areas to address in order to sustain and advance — Where are we?

Track/Report

Adapt/Update

Transition to Implementation — Specify action steps, accountabilities, and resources — Specifics to carry out plan and estimate plan impact — How do we execute?

Organizational Direction — Affirm mission, values; establish vision and overall strategy — High-level direction to pursue — Where should we be going?

Strategy Formulation — Develop goals, metrics, and initiatives — Key desired outcomes and priority activities — How do we get there?

vision, values, and key strategies for the organization. Strategy formulation establishes goals, objectives, and major initiatives for the organization. The purpose of stages 2 and 3 of the planning process is to determine what broad future direction is possible and desirable and what future scope of services and position the organization will strive to achieve.

The fourth stage is implementation planning—how do we get there? This stage involves identifying the actions needed to implement the plan. Key activities include mapping out the tasks to accomplish the goals and objectives, setting a schedule, determining priorities, and allocating resources to ensure implementation. Implementation should begin as soon as possible after completion of the plan, if not during the final stage. Teams should ensure that commitment to ongoing monitoring of plan implementation and completion of periodic updates and revisions, as needed, are in place prior to finalizing the plan. Each stage of the planning process is discussed in detail in the following chapters.

BUT WHY STRATEGIC PLANNING?

Understanding Primary Criticisms

As referenced in the opening of this chapter, not all commentators agree that strategic planning is an effective way to set good strategy. Several criticisms and possible pitfalls commonly arise (the next section comprises a list of the latter), but three primary criticisms of strategic planning prevail:

1. It relies on past or current conditions and performance as relevant predictors of the future.
2. It yields a static output that is unable to account for dynamic realities.
3. The formality and prescriptiveness of the process may actually hinder the thoughtful reflection and forward-looking creative thinking that is critical to good strategy.

Note that none of the primary criticisms of planning actually preclude it from being a useful means to good strategy. Criticisms assume that certain attributes of planning are inherent or immutable, and that potential problems with some planning processes can be generalized to discredit the whole of strategic planning. As evinced in part in the following chapter and elaborated on in later chapters, these assumptions are not necessarily valid.

For example, consider the first of the primary criticisms noted previously—reliance on the past to predict the future. Yes, the practice of scanning the environment and the organization's performance and position requires using historical data. However, in a well-conceived strategic planning process, findings from analysis are not intended to be used as a basis to project forward. Rather, as described in chapter 6, historical data are just one input that must be contextualized based on assumptions about the future environment. This criticism falsely assumes that because planning *could* solely rely on past information to make decisions about the future, then it must necessarily do so, or that it could not be otherwise balanced by incorporation of future-oriented thinking.

The second criticism implies that strategic plans are not effective guides once the environment shifts or the organization undergoes change. This inference is logical if the planning process ended after strategy formulation and development of initial action plans; however, as described in chapters 9 and 10, an effective planning process establishes and activates a continuous implementation and plan management approach that ensures ongoing review and updates. These activities are typically sufficient to minimize the risk of plans becoming gradually less relevant and thus less useful over time.

The third criticism is more philosophical. It suggests that formal structures impede originality and therefore undermine strategic thinking. However, every artist works in a particular medium or media. Artists are constrained in some ways by the guidelines and tools of the chosen medium, but nonetheless express inspiration and imagination. A well-structured strategic planning process, as described in the remainder of this book, functions much like these guidelines and tools. It provides a framework to gather information, input, and insight supporting the development and implementation of effective strategy. Absent such a structure, an organization could theoretically get lucky, creating and executing great strategies, but it will be following a far riskier path that can more easily lead it astray.

Therefore, organizational leaders should focus on getting the strategic planning process right, not skipping it. While modifications to the comprehensive strategic planning process that this chapter previously outlined can be made, the fundamental logic behind and core steps of the planning approach should remain. Despite the ongoing debate over the efficacy and methods of strategic planning, it remains the most relevant means to develop strategy. Too often, leaders who avoid strategic planning also bypass strategic thinking.

Even so, linking strategic planning to good strategy and specific organizational success is difficult (Ginter, Duncan, and Swayne 2013; Kaissi and Begun 2008), though scholars do acknowledge that strategic planning adds value to organizations: "By planning and evolving to meet expected changes head on, organizations have a better chance of survival" (Bellenfant and Nelson 2016, 1). Because strategic planning requires examining functionality and sustainability, it improves awareness of an organization's relative strengths and weaknesses. This enhanced awareness generates focus, which alone can have a positive impact on organizational performance and thus improve chances of long-term survival. Nonetheless, pinpointing specific effects of strategic planning is challenging, and success will depend on and vary with managerial, environmental, and organizational factors (Taiwo and Idunnu 2010).

The authors of this book fully acknowledge that strategic planning has limitations and is not a foolproof way to create effective strategy. Further, we reiterate the merit in understanding and purposefully addressing key criticisms. In fact, subsequent chapters dedicated to each of the four stages of the strategic planning approach specifically identify how planning can go wrong and how to be aware of and proactively correct for such challenges.

Understanding Common Pitfalls

The previously mentioned primary criticisms are the basis of many common problems faced in strategic planning, but several others are worth noting, as they often leave leaders jaded about the value of such planning.

Failing to Involve the Appropriate People
Sometimes too many stakeholders are involved; sometimes too few. Sometimes the number of participants is fine, but those involved are

not necessarily the "right" people. Thoughtful involvement of the right type and mix of internal and external stakeholders is essential to both strategy development and successful implementation.

Conducting Strategic Planning Independent of Financial Planning

If financial considerations are excluded from the strategic plan, strategies may never become a reality. Sound strategic planning will explicitly incorporate financial realities and test the financial reasonableness of executing an identified strategic approach.

Falling Prey to Analysis Paralysis

The fast-paced healthcare market demands that provider organizations respond to opportunities and threats without extensive delays. As such, squandering time by endlessly analyzing and reanalyzing data in the hopes of more accurate baselines or forecasts works against the intent of planning: to prepare for and effectively respond to change.

Not Addressing the Critical Issues

Planning teams may avoid the most pressing issues because they are too difficult to discuss or address. In addition, planning teams may identify a litany of issues but not subsequently refine the list to those that are most critical. If leadership is not prepared to address key issues or to actively ensure a sense of focus, strategic planning can ignore or overlook the most threatening challenges and potentially powerful opportunities.

Failing to Achieve Consensus

Even an objectively great strategic plan cannot succeed unless it is strongly supported by those responsible for its execution. Leadership and strategic plan facilitators must purposefully build this support and cannot ignore disagreements or even a lack of strong, visible consensus on key plan components. Organizational leaders must repeatedly test for broad agreement and generate enthusiasm about the plan while it is being developed.

Ignoring Resistance to Change

Like the inability to tackle what is truly critical or build appropriate consensus, ignoring resistance to change will have detrimental long-term consequences. The types and degree of change proposed in a plan must be seen by all involved as necessary to future organizational success. Organizational leaders must swiftly and directly address persistent opposition to change to avoid devastating effects, including significant delays, wasting of time and resources, and even complete derailment of progress.

Ineffectively Transitioning from Planning to Execution

Failure to execute is both common and highly detrimental. An organization cannot simply identify goals and objectives and assume that identification will result in implementation. Rather, a purposeful and thorough transition from planning to execution must occur that clearly establishes accountabilities and the action steps that create a path forward. Without such care, the day-to-day operational crises that inevitably arise will consume staff and leaders, leaving execution of strategy an afterthought. Further, goals and objectives must be precise and measurable enough to create individual accountability and make success or failure obvious.

Understanding Key Benefits

Chapter 2 is dedicated to realizing the benefits of strategic planning, but a high-level summary of the advantages of strategic planning is helpful as well. C. Davis Fogg (2010) suggests the following benefits of strategic planning:

- It secures the future for the organization and its leaders by crafting a viable future business.
- It provides a road map, direction, and focus for the organization's future—where it wants to go and the routes to get there. It lets each part of the organization align

its activities with the direction of the corporation in a continuous process.

- It sets priorities for crucial strategic tasks, including complex, pressing issues such as lack of direction and growth, lack of profitability, and organizational ineffectiveness—issues that everybody talks and knows about yet remain unaddressed.
- It allocates resources available for growth and change to the programs and activities with the highest potential payoff.
- It establishes measures of success so that the progress of the organization and individuals can be gauged. Knowing where one stands is a fundamental business and human need.
- It gathers input and ideas from all parts of the organization on what can be done to ensure future success and eliminate barriers to that success, following the old adage that two (or ten, or a hundred, or a thousand) heads are better than one.
- It generates commitment to implementing the plan by involving all parts of the organization in the plan's development.
- It coordinates the actions of diverse and separate parts of the organization into unified programs to accomplish objectives.

Fogg (2010, 76) further notes that "when all is said and done, employees also recognize what's in it for them personally: the resources to do what they want if they plan; a more secure future if the organization plans well and does well; financial rewards if they make themselves heroes as a result of the process; recognition by their peers and superiors if they succeed; and, of course, the inverse of all the above if they fail."

Ginter, Duncan, and Swayne (2013) believe that the three stages of strategic management—strategic thinking, strategic planning, and strategic momentum—provide many benefits, including

- tying the organization together with a common sense of purpose and shared values;
- improving financial performance in many cases;
- providing the organization with a clear self-concept, specific goals, and guidance and consistency in decision making;
- helping managers understand the present, think about the future, and recognize the signals that suggest change;
- requiring managers to communicate both vertically and horizontally;
- improving overall coordination in the organization; and
- encouraging innovation and change in the organization to meet the needs of dynamic situations.

For many organizations the true value of strategic planning lies in the process, not the plan. In fact, as D. A. Nadler (1994) points out, most plans have a fast rate of depreciation; by the time they're done, they're obsolete. Thus, much of the value of planning isn't the actual plan, but rather the shared learning, shared frame of reference, and shared context for decision making.

Indeed, changes that influence a strategic plan may occur daily, and new ideas may surface once the plan is complete. A successful strategic plan enables providers to establish a consistent, well-articulated direction for the future. However, it is also a living document that teams must monitor and revise to meet the anticipated and unanticipated needs of the organization and the market, whether changes occur in clinical services, managed care, integrated delivery, payment models, healthcare reform, systems development, technological advances, or other arenas.

STRATEGIC PLANNING IN HEALTHCARE

Compared to organizations in other major sectors of the economy, healthcare provider organizations historically survived using less formalized planning approaches. Prior to the 1970s, healthcare provider organizations were predominately independent and not-for-profit, and healthcare planning was usually conducted on a local or regional basis by state, county, or municipal governments. Though formally introduced in the early 1970s, healthcare organizations used strategic planning only sporadically, and their focus remained on better identifying and meeting community needs rather than more modern competitive objectives.

As illustrated in exhibit 1.2, government regulation became more prominent in healthcare in the late 1970s. Healthcare organizations undertook planning efforts in part to address new regulatory barriers, but the fee-for-service system continued to ensure a steady revenue stream. As such, when healthcare organizations engaged in strategic planning, the effort often focused on creating physical capacity to accommodate more and more volume, with the prevailing notion being that "if you build it, they will come." The 1980s brought privatization and corporatization to the healthcare sector. Hospitals were consolidated into systems, and healthcare corporations began to enter and organize other healthcare-related fields. The 1990s and early 2000s were characterized by the chaos of managed care and competition among providers who had previously been collegial. Strategic planning conducted at this time heavily emphasized maximizing reimbursement.

As the central principles of broader healthcare reform took shape in the early twenty-first century, it started to become clear that healthcare organizations would have to do more with less. This fact remains true today and will likely hold, regardless of future political changes, because some certainties are clear. Healthcare costs have grown at rates above general inflation, creating growing burdens on employers, governments, and individuals. The population will

Exhibit 1.2: A History of Healthcare Strategic Planning

	1960s	1970s	1980s	1990s	Early 2000s	2010+
Environment	Medicare and Medicaid established Fee-for-service (FFS) Cost-plus reimbursement	FFS Federal regulation Growing hospital expenses and profits	Hospital system formation Diagnosis-related groups (DRGs) Capitation	Growing competition Expansion of managed care First-generation federal health reform proposed	Pay-for-performance (P4P) State-based health reform Major pharma and technology advancements	Emergence of value-based payment Reduced hospital-centricity Performance data transparency
Strategic planning focus	Little need; not widely used Meeting community needs	Adding capacity; building hospitals	Consolidating hospitals Containing costs	Maximizing reimbursement Protecting territory and margins	Optimizing payer mix Maximizing P4P incentives Appealing directly to consumers	Creating scale Integrating care delivery Demonstrating quality and cost performance

continue to age. Patient care that is coordinated and that produces objectively higher-quality outcomes will be rewarded. The shortage of physicians, nurses, and other care professionals will not go away.

As a result, providers across the country are examining their current and future role in an era when quality, consumer orientation, cost competitiveness, scale and scope, and integration will move to the forefront of strategic priorities. Many may need a strategic overhaul to orient the organization to the realities of a new era in healthcare delivery and financing. Providers will be challenged to innovate across all domains, and differentiation will require proactive development of an array of new competencies for clinicians and business leaders. Transformational information technology and competition from entrepreneurs outside of healthcare as well as both for-profit provider and financing entities will add additional complexity to the healthcare landscape. Healthcare provider organizations with thoughtful, sound strategic plans will be best positioned to adapt with contingency plans as change emerges.

Evolution of Healthcare Strategic Planning

The first-generation healthcare strategic planning approach that was developed in the 1970s is clearly much less relevant in today's complex environment. As a result, the application of strategic planning in healthcare organizations today differs from that of the past in five critical ways:

1. Healthcare is changing at an unprecedentedly fast pace. This pace presses organizational leaders to conduct strategic planning in a more dynamic fashion.
2. The competitive environment is much more intense than at any time in the past. The number of competitors, the increasing for-profit influence in healthcare delivery, the decline of geographic barriers to competition as a result of the Internet, and other less significant factors raise the

competitive stakes and force strategic planning to be more externally focused and fluid.

3. Healthcare organizations have grown into vast multientity systems. The emergence of systems, especially in the past five to ten years, has ratcheted up the complexity of strategic planning.

4. Intense competition and new payment models have destabilized the financial underpinning of healthcare delivery. When organizations are operating in an environment of increasing financial risk and uncertainty, strategic planning needs to be linked more clearly to financial planning and contribute more directly to financial performance.

5. The time frame in which to act and generate results is tightening. Strategic planning must address near-term pressures while still directing organizations toward long-term targets.

However, even if healthcare strategic planning has become much more sophisticated, planning approaches must continue to evolve to address emerging and dynamic challenges affecting all aspects of healthcare delivery and financing.

Ensuring Applicability of Strategic Planning in Healthcare

Much strategic planning and strategy for healthcare organizations has emphasized operational effectiveness—doing the same things as peers and competitors but doing it better (that is, with higher quality or more efficiently) as opposed to true competitive differentiation. However, some strategy experts (Porter 1996) assert that operational effectiveness is not strategy, largely because operational effectiveness does not satisfy several of the previously mentioned criteria for effective strategy: namely, sustainability, competitive advantages, and direction. Organizational leaders often express a similar sentiment when they say, "Achieving operational effectiveness is a given."

Although typical business practices in the for-profit and private sectors have been advocated as applicable to healthcare, there are legitimate questions about the validity of assuming that business paradigms are appropriate in healthcare (Ginter, Duncan, and Swayne 2013). In addition to, and in some ways as the result of being a primarily not-for-profit and mission-driven field, healthcare is different from other fields in key ways that may mitigate the applicability of standard business practices, including the following:

- Healthcare services are not a typical product and cannot be standardized.
- It is difficult for users to predict when they will need healthcare or how much they might need.
- Unpredictable needs result in unpredictable costs and little price transparency, making it hard for consumers to make decisions based on value.
- The user is not the payer for most of the cost, though high-deductible health plans are reducing this dynamic.
- Information asymmetry persists, as the provider of services has knowledge and expertise that the user would not reasonably have, even with access to online medical information.
- Physicians are key decision makers but may not be part of the healthcare organization nor subject to the same set of incentives.
- Providers routinely address serious health issues (some are life and death) that elevate individual and societal expectations beyond those in a simple commercial transaction.
- Healthcare organizations are subject to a unique set of regulations:

- They may not be able to divest of a service even if it is not profitable.
- They can only "choose" customers to a limited degree.
- They are subject to significant governmental and other regulatory bodies, mandates, and compliance requirements.

Ginter, Duncan, and Swayne (2013) summarize the implications of these unique traits on healthcare providers with regard to strategic planning and strategy:

- Some strategic alternatives available to nonhealthcare organizations may not be realistic for many healthcare organizations.
- Healthcare organizations have unique cultures that influence the style of and participation in strategic planning.
- Healthcare has always been subject to considerable outside control.
- Society and its values place special demands on healthcare organizations.

These factors clearly call for healthcare providers to develop a customized approach to strategic planning that accounts for its distinctive qualities—a process that, to an extent, has begun to occur and will continue to evolve with time. The sector's uniqueness does not, however, discredit the relevance of strategy-related business practices in general. In fact, the type of healthcare sector changes under way, as well as the fast pace and amplitude of changes, may suggest that strategic business practices from other industries may actually be more relevant to healthcare in the future. In any case, healthcare sector transformation necessitates healthcare organizations' adoption of sophisticated strategic planning and management practices in order to adapt and thrive in the future.

REFERENCES

Beckham, J. D. 2016. *What Good Strategy Is.* Southeastern Institute for Health Care Strategy and Innovation. Published July 29. www.hcstrategyinnovation.com/assets/WhatGoodStrategyIs.pdf.
———. 2000. "Strategy: What It Is, How It Works, Why It Fails." *Health Forum Journal* 43 (6): 55–59.

Bellenfant, W., and M. J. Nelson. 2016. "Improving Performance Through Execution of Strategy." Financial Resource Group. Accessed November 28. http://frgroup.net/articles/article_strategic_planning.pdf.

Campbell, A. B. 1993. "Strategic Planning in Health Care: Methods and Applications." *Quality Management in Health Care* 1 (4): 12–23.

Eisenhardt, K. M. 1999. "Strategy as Strategic Decision Making." *Sloan Management Review* 40 (3): 65–72.

Evashwick, C. J., and W. T. Evashwick. 1988. "The Fine Art of Strategic Planning." *Provider* 14 (4): 4–6.

Fogg, C. D. 2010. *Team-Based Strategic Planning: A Complete Guide to Structuring, Facilitating, and Implementing the Process.* No place: CreateSpace Independent Publishing Platform.

Ginter, P. M., W. J. Duncan, and L. E. Swayne. 2013. *Strategic Management of Health Care Organizations*, 7th ed. San Francisco: Jossey-Bass.

Hamel, G., and C. K. Prahalad. 1989. "Strategic Intent." *Harvard Business Review*, May–June, 63–76.

Kaissi, A. A., and J. W. Begun. 2008. "Strategic Planning Processes and Hospital Financial Performance." *Journal of Healthcare Management* 53 (3): 197–208.

Martin, R. L. 2014. "The Big Lie of Strategic Planning." *Harvard Business Review*, January–February, 3–8.

Mintzberg, H. 1994. "The Fall and Rise of Strategic Planning." *Harvard Business Review*, January–February, 107–13.

————. 1978. "Patterns in Strategy Formation." *Management Science* 24 (9): 934–48.

Mintzberg, H., B. Ahlstrand, and J. Lampel. 1998. *Strategy Safari: A Guided Tour Through the Wilds of Strategic Management.* New York: Free Press.

Nadler, D. A. 1994. "Collaborative Strategic Thinking." *Planning Review* 22 (5): 30–44.

Porter, M. E. 1998. *Competitive Advantage: Creating and Sustaining Superior Performance*, 2nd ed. New York: Free Press.

————. 1996. "What Is Strategy?" *Harvard Business Review*, November–December, 61–78.

————. 1979. "How Competitive Forces Shape Strategy." *Harvard Business Review*, March, 137–45.

Rumelt, R. 2011a. *Good Strategy, Bad Strategy: The Difference and Why It Matters.* New York: Crown Business.

————. 2011b. "The Perils of Bad Strategy." *McKinsey Quarterly*, June, 30–39.

Simyar, F., J. Lloyd-Jones, and J. Caro. 1988. "Strategic Management: A Proposed Framework for the Health Care Industry." In *Strategic Management in the Health Care Sector: Toward the Year 2000*, edited by F. Simyar and J. Lloyd-Jones, 6–17. Englewood Cliffs, NJ: Prentice Hall.

Skinner, W. 1969. "Manufacturing—Missing Link in Corporate Strategy." *Harvard Business Review*, May, 136–45.

Sorkin, D. L., N. B. Ferris, and J. Hudak. 1984. *Strategies for Cities and Counties: A Strategic Planning Guide.* Washington, DC: Public Technology, Inc.

Taiwo, A. S., and F. O. Idunnu. 2010. "Impact of Strategic Planning on Organizational Performance and Survival." *Research Journal of Business Management* 4 (1): 73–82.

Benefits of Strategic Planning

Good fortune is what happens when opportunity meets
with planning.

—Thomas Edison

The true measure of your worth includes all the benefits
others have gained from your success.

—Cullen Hightower

Why should an organization carry out strategic planning? What
benefits can be expected from this effort? How can the strategic planning process be structured and managed to maximize the likelihood
that benefits will be realized? These and other important questions
will be addressed in this chapter.

Unfortunately, while there may be a sound basis for conducting
strategic planning, strategic plans regularly fail to achieve their promise. Survey results in healthcare and nonhealthcare literature alike
reveal that many organizations struggle with realizing the benefits of
strategic planning. Extensive surveys of the literature on this subject
yield decidedly mixed results depending on how strategic planning
is defined and what specific benefits are under consideration.

The authors of this book routinely survey healthcare provider
organizational leadership on this topic and find that leaders feel that
benefit realization does not match up to the quality of the plans

developed and the planning processes. Respondents indicate that despite very effective strategic planning processes, strong plans, and reasonably good implementation, the results achieved (i.e., benefits) did not meet expectations.

Though there are likely many reasons underlying these results, we attribute these findings primarily to a lack of clarity in and visibility of the benefits sought from the outset and throughout the planning process. Some organizations plunge into strategic planning without identifying what may be gained through the process (see chapter 3 on the organization of the preplanning process for recommendations on avoiding this particular pitfall). Some groups identify so many expected outcomes that it is difficult to interpret or remember the main purposes. Others provide only vague expectations, so stakeholders are not really sure of the purposes or the potential benefits. Still others get off to a clear, good start, but then veer off course during the process through inadequate, inconsistent, or contradictory communications about intended benefits.

The remainder of this chapter provides guidance on identifying potential benefits as well as how to promote realization of these benefits.

IDENTIFYING STRATEGIC PLANNING BENEFITS

Substantive (i.e., non-process-related) strategic planning benefits can be identified at the outset and pursued throughout the planning process. These benefits should fall into one or more of four categories:

1. Product and market improvement
2. Financial improvement
3. Operational improvement
4. Community needs realization

The following sections review each category of benefit and describe what is desirable and possible to achieve.

Product and Market Improvement

Historically, strategic planning has been oriented toward achieving product and market benefits. Larger service areas, higher market shares, more comprehensive products and services, and, recently, improved linkages among services have formed the core of healthcare strategic planning's concerns (see exhibit 2.1). Relative to other areas of potential benefits, product and market improvement has been addressed fairly well by healthcare organizations. However, many organizations are reevaluating traditional product and market strategies and metrics as they move from fee-for-service to fee-for-value and shift to bundled and risk-based payments and population health management.

Market or service area. Every healthcare organization's strategic plan is at least somewhat focused on protection, if not expansion, of its market or service area. Even in the most rural areas and certainly in all urban and suburban areas, the geographical area primarily served by the organization is of interest to competitors and is increasingly at risk. Because of the increasingly competitive nature of healthcare, offensive strategies that target new geographical markets are quite common. Despite the primacy of this topic, strategic planning efforts have achieved mixed results regarding growth and defense of service areas. Often, the populations in certain markets are shared among providers. Sharing populations is likely to become less common with the shift toward population health management and as taking responsibility (clinical and financial) for a clearly defined group of people becomes more prevalent.

Market share. Equally important are strategies to increase existing market shares. Most strategic plans conclude that market share increases are desirable and feasible, particularly as utilization rates are anticipated to decrease through better population health management. In the majority of cases, such conclusions and related initiatives do lead to increased shares, at least for some services if not overall.

Exhibit 2.1: What Product or Market Benefits Can and Should Be Achieved?

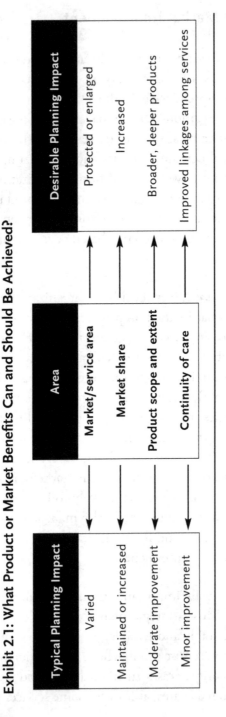

Typical Planning Impact	Area	Desirable Planning Impact
Varied	Market/service area	Protected or enlarged
Maintained or increased	Market share	Increased
Moderate improvement	Product scope and extent	Broader, deeper products
Minor improvement	Continuity of care	Improved linkages among services

© 2017 Veralon Partners Inc.

Readers should also note that, in connection with the defined population concept, market share targets for some provider organizations may also include share of covered lives in addition to traditional market share for inpatient or outpatient services. Given its newness as a focus area in strategic planning, there are challenges in establishing accurate baselines and appropriate growth targets for share of covered lives, and the extent to which desired results are actually achieved remains unclear.

Product scope and extent. Most healthcare providers now recognize that the growth of products (i.e., programs, services) can no longer be managed on an ad hoc basis or exclusively in an opportunistic manner. Rather, leadership teams must explicitly formulate a focused and systematic approach in order to appropriately broaden and deepen service offerings and to better organize and integrate the overall product portfolio. Further, and as a result of changing sector norms and consumer expectations, the strategic plans of healthcare organizations increasingly feature recommendations for development and growth that extend beyond acute care, and in some instances, beyond healthcare services delivery (e.g., they may include a payer function). Exhibit 2.2 presents a framework for identifying and organizing the potential range of products and competencies offered by health systems today. The framework also illustrates how services and programs should interrelate and provides context on the relationships, functions, and expectations that shape a modern health system's product portfolio. As a result of the incorporation of relatively novel functions and the associated complexity of aggregating and managing a broader array of products, realization of strategic planning benefits in this domain is uneven across health systems to date.

Continuity of care. Related to the broadened and evolving definition of product scope and extent is the consideration of how services and programs in a health system's portfolio are coordinated and managed to ensure continuity of care. Continuity of care is basically

Exhibit 2.2: Modern Healthcare System Product Scope Framework

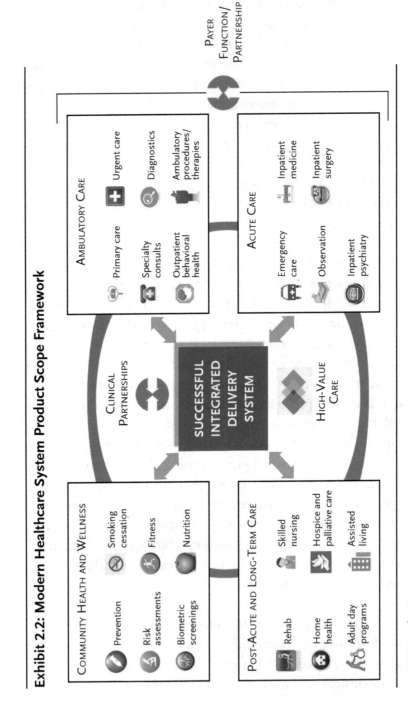

© 2017 Veralon Partners Inc.

a second-generation result of integrated care delivery, and many healthcare organizations now attempt to address continuity and coordination of services across care settings and continua as part of the strategic planning process. Though care continuity is not novel for organizations with a historic commitment to vertical integration, or to those early adopters of population health management principles, its benefits are nonetheless hard to achieve. Effective coordination of care depends on the ability to offer a broad range of services that are both owned and affiliated, as well as clear linkages among and seamless transitions across services. Healthcare leaders increasingly appreciate that developing capabilities and capitalizing on the potential benefits of integrated delivery take time, and thus continuity of care is an increasingly common and important modern strategic planning topic.

Financial Benefits

This category of likely substantive benefit is probably the most obvious and is applicable to all healthcare organizations; however, realization of financial benefits has been mixed at best. Exhibit 2.3 identifies four general areas of financial benefit along with the historically most prevalent outcome versus the desired planning impact. Healthcare organizations can better achieve financial benefits if they effectively involve financial leadership and integrate financial planning into the process.

Operating margin. Few, if any, healthcare organizations have such a high operating margin that they can ignore the need to maintain or increase it. For many organizations today, increasing the operating margin is a primary goal of strategic planning. Unfortunately, strategic plans often identify initiatives that require significant operating resources to execute, which can cut into the margin. In addition, operating margins can suffer when healthcare organizations try to balance volume optimization under fee-for-service arrangements with

Exhibit 2.3: What Financial Benefits Can and Should Be Achieved?

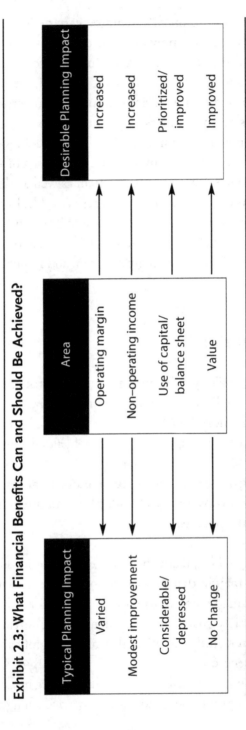

Typical Planning Impact	Area	Desirable Planning Impact
Varied	Operating margin	Increased
Modest improvement	Non–operating income	Increased
Considerable/ depressed	Use of capital/ balance sheet	Prioritized/ improved
No change	Value	Improved

population health management and reduced utilization in a value-based payment environment. Finally, some healthcare organization strategic plans are still too oriented toward "meeting community needs" without an eye toward sustainability, or leadership generates strategic plans to satisfy internal constituents without appropriate regard for the impact on financial performance generally. As a result of all these factors, and consistent with the results of the literature on strategic planning, plans are just as likely to decrease operating margin as they are to increase it.

Non–operating income. This issue has not been a high priority for many healthcare organizations until fairly recently. However, the bull market of the 1990s and secondary rapid growth spurt in the stock market in the early twenty-first century raised the profile of this issue considerably. In addition to sound investment management, an increasing number of healthcare organizations have targeted philanthropy as a high-priority strategy. Such organizations have developed sophisticated, comprehensive fundraising programs and have generated significant non–operating income to fund capital projects, as seed money for clinical program investment, and to build endowments. A small number of organizations have developed large-scale clinical research enterprises, innovation centers, consulting practices, and other ventures unrelated to patient care to tap into additional non–operating income sources. Though considered commonplace today, diversification away from the core healthcare business can be difficult and should be approached cautiously.

Access to capital; balance sheet indicators. Another typical reason for commencing strategic planning is to help support or rationalize capital-intensive facilities, technology, or other investments. In fact, strategic planning is commonly used outside of healthcare for the purpose of making difficult choices among capital investment alternatives, and some healthcare organizations use strategic planning in a similar manner. Unfortunately, even today, some strategic plans lead to capital consumption without appropriate regard for the downstream financial impact.

Further, only rarely, despite the increasingly difficult financial climate in healthcare, is improvement of the balance sheet stated as a desired strategic planning outcome. Given the frequent failure to improve operating margin, it is understandable that the balance sheet can often deteriorate as a result of strategic planning. Nonetheless, few organizations can afford to see their balance sheets suffer, even as a result of important projects. Balance sheet management has not been a priority in the planning process among nonfinancially oriented healthcare executives and boards, but there is a positive and growing trend toward accurately estimating and accounting for the balance sheet impact of strategic planning.

Value. The high and rising cost of healthcare in the United States has brought the concept of value to the forefront in healthcare strategic planning. Value is created when the quality (e.g., clinical outcomes, consumer satisfaction) derived from healthcare delivery exceeds the cost (or price). Readers should note that many healthcare providers are broadening their scopes of interest from the value of a procedure, hospital stay, or visit to the value across an episode of care (e.g., bundled payments) or across all care received by a given patient population (e.g., accountable care organizations [ACOs], risk sharing). Value often tops the list of healthcare organizations' critical issues today and thus is becoming a standard strategic planning priority.

Case Example: Strategic Planning Facilitates Realization of Financial Benefit for a Large, Integrated Health System in the Midwest

Amid financial and organizational uncertainty associated with a significant leadership transition, a billion-dollar integrated delivery system based in the Midwest—consisting of several acute care hospitals, a large employed medical group, an expansive network of ambulatory and extended care services, an ACO, and a health plan—embraced strategic planning as a means to structure organizational turnaround efforts and achieve financial results in all four areas described in exhibit 2.3.

Championed by a new and stabilized executive team, the strategic planning process yielded focused growth strategies aimed at restoring and securing financial health. The year after plan completion, the health system achieved an operating margin of approximately 5 percent. In addition, the plan called for extensive modernization of its philanthropy program, which boosted non–operating income. These improvements allowed the system to undertake its largest capital investment in nearly a decade the following year, setting in motion growth initiatives that should reap significant dividends in the years to come.

In addition to targeted efforts to bolster the operating margin and cultivate new sources of non–operating income, the strategic plan emphasized differentiating based on value. Value-driven strategies focused on maximizing the ACO to reduce costs and improve quality for a defined population and on partnering with a number of community health agencies to manage the costs of caring for residents in more rural, outlying service area regions.

Operational Benefits

In contrast to financial benefit, operational benefit tends to be an under recognized and underappreciated category. In addition, some planners make the error of avoiding operational benefit because they believe operational concerns are not strategic. Yet, operational benefit is of strategic importance to nearly all healthcare organizations, and many areas in this category will increase in strategic importance over the next decade. Leaders can realize tremendous strategic improvement by including operational improvement in strategic planning. To effectively address operational improvement in strategic planning, the planning team must elevate the focus to high-level areas rather than get dragged into debates over minor operational issues.

Exhibit 2.4 identifies four general areas of operational improvement benefits, along with the historically most prevalent outcome versus the desired planning impact.

Patient satisfaction. In a service sector such as healthcare, few topics are as important to success as satisfied and engaged customers. Yet, customer satisfaction was not a major concern of healthcare organizations until the competitive era emerged in the 1990s and early 2000s, brought on by the financial uncertainties of managed care and cemented by direct-to-consumer advertising. Now, with increased visibility and availability of comparative healthcare organization information, customer satisfaction has moved from the background to the foreground in competitive—and, therefore, strategic—importance.

The emergence of patient-centered care delivery models and consumer-oriented services design are evidence of provider organizations' recognition of this development. Whether the patient satisfaction metrics proposed by sector experts and used by healthcare organization leadership teams today truly reflect patient and family satisfaction with healthcare services is unclear, but the ubiquitous presence of these metrics on health system and hospital scorecards emphasizes the awareness and criticality of this area. Plans that do not acknowledge (or better yet comprehensively address) this area are likely to fall short of the mark in terms of the realization of key benefits.

Quality. Healthcare quality was in a position similar to that of customer satisfaction until the late 1990s—it was a major concern of the general public but not necessarily of healthcare organizations. Awareness and action were incited by the publication of the first Institute of Medicine report on medical errors (1999), which highlighted significant safety and general quality-of-care issues. Efforts to measure consistently and to publicize healthcare quality data have taken hold, and competing on quality level is considered a strategic imperative.

Exhibit 2.4: What Operational Benefits Can and Should Be Achieved?

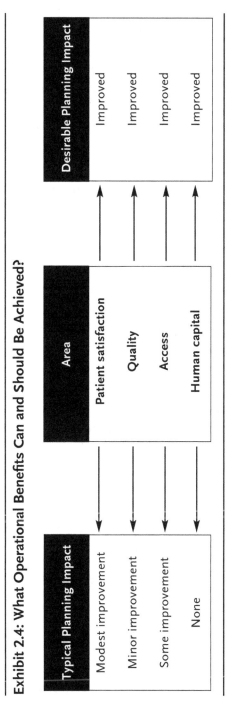

Typical Planning Impact	Area	Desirable Planning Impact
Modest improvement	Patient satisfaction	Improved
Minor improvement	Quality	Improved
Some improvement	Access	Improved
None	Human capital	Improved

© 2017 Veralon Partners Inc.

Significant advances in measuring and improving healthcare quality have been made in the last decade, specifically on structure and process measures. Improving performance on outcomes measures has proven more challenging for healthcare organizations and will be even more crucial as a greater proportion of provider reimbursement is tied to demonstrating value. Tremendous gains in quality are likely to emerge over the next decade. Strategic plans need to emphasize improved performance on the more transformational measures of outcome that will almost certainly be key factors in differentiating healthcare organizations in the future.

Access. The majority of healthcare consumers access services in community settings, yet most health systems remain primarily oriented to the business of the hospital. The proven importance of a high-functioning primary care network to overall health system sustainability—and to managing population health—support the notion that access to care should be a central strategic concern. Linked to the broader consumerism movement, convenience and all facets of accessibility, including virtual access, have become paramount issues.

Nearly all organizations face challenges in organizing the right suite of coordinated outpatient and physician services in the right places. Because of the magnitude of problems in this area, its large and growing importance as a centerpiece of state and national reform initiatives, and the capital and incremental operating expenditures required to address these issues, this topic has been the priority of many strategic planners in the past few years, with modest success to date and much more needed in the future.

Human capital. The centrality of employees and physicians to the success of healthcare organizations has long been acknowledged, but effectively harnessing human capital still eludes even the best provider organizations. Fierce competition to recruit clinicians makes setting high expectations difficult, but problems with meaningful alignment and engagement represent the real hurdle. Despite the significance of this issue, it is on the big-picture strategic agenda of only a handful of organizations; most expect the human resources department and operations leaders to do the heavy lifting. As a result, it is often ignored in the strategic planning process, even though the magnitude of the challenge, its systemic nature, and its highest-order strategic implications suggest otherwise. An effective strategic planning process should highlight the potential competitive differentiation that a focus on human capital can yield by calling for initiatives to better align, engage, and leverage talent across the healthcare delivery enterprise.

Case Example: UW Health's Focus on Realizing Operational Benefits

Like many first- and second-generation integrated delivery systems, the University of Wisconsin's health system, UW Health, has done much to streamline operations and make them more patient centric. UW Health has largely achieved its primary goals of growth and financial health in the course of its strategic planning and execution over the last 15 years. In the update of its strategic plan in 2013, while growth and financial health remained important priorities, of equal or possibly greater importance was operational integration and improvement.

In 2013, UW Health consisted of a university hospital, large multispecialty physician group, and a health plan. It operated primarily in Madison, Wisconsin, and the surrounding region. The hospital and physician group were separate, though related, organizations and as independent entities did not always mesh well together for the patients they jointly served. To make a great leap forward in providing value-based care, the highest priority in the 2013 strategic plan for the umbrella organization, UW Health, was to make integration a reality. The initial result of this was the merger of the hospital and physician group in 2015.

This merger enabled the organization to undertake important strategic initiatives to improve quality and care delivery throughout UW Health. The initial efforts in patient and family-centered care, begun a few years earlier, were greatly expanded to all parts of the organization, with a particular focus on the emergency department. Continuous quality improvement was formalized as the "UW Way" through physician and administrative leader dyads. A major push was made to standardize all primary care to meet the requirements of patient-centered medical homes. The goal to make UW Health the best workplace and academic environment possible also received significant attention over the past few years through workforce planning, training and integration, formalized leadership training, and team-based care delivery models. As a result, quality and patient satisfaction scores have risen significantly.

Community Benefits

Not-for-profit healthcare organizations typically have focused on and attempted to demonstrate community benefits as part of their strategic plan. Often, however, and increasingly so, this area of benefit is "talked up" more than it is actually addressed, even though not-for-profits are required to prioritize and be responsive to the needs of the communities they serve. In fact, there have been challenges to the tax-exempt status of health systems based in part on their failure to demonstrate meaningful community benefit.

For many modern healthcare organizations, there is a growing disconnect between their community service mission and the actual attention and resources devoted to making it a reality. This gap is, at least in part, because healthcare organizations have become larger, more complex businesses serving broad areas. Thus they are more distant and detached from the communities that originally spawned them. Though the ways in which healthcare organizations can generate community benefit and the types of community benefit sought have evolved, this area represents an instance in which recalling a more traditional, historically held mind-set may actually help organizations succeed in the future.

Exhibit 2.5 identifies four general areas of community benefits, along with the most prevalent outcome historically versus the desired planning impact.

Needed services provided. Identifying community needs and ensuring that the needed care is provided were the primary concerns of healthcare strategic planning on inception and, appropriately, remain important today. Providing needed services is probably the community benefit that healthcare organizations most effectively realize, in part because healthcare provider competition has traditionally been focused on service breadth and depth, thus heightening the relevance of pursuing this benefit.

Community health improvement. Many healthcare organizations have made community health improvement the centerpiece of their mission statements. Periodically, this area has been an important strategic concern. On a more frequent basis, it has been given lip service and addressed, if at all, indirectly. Especially for not-for-profits, contributing to community health improvement should be a key element of community benefit. Difficulties in having a measurable, population-level impact and the inherent conflict of a field traditionally oriented to treating the sick in an episodic way hinder constructive efforts. However, health systems are well positioned to support these efforts through education, wellness, and outreach efforts, often for a relatively low cost. In addition, the importance of, and in many ways accountability for, community health improvement has been given a boost by the increasing emphasis on broader accountability for the care of a population (see the following section titled "Population health management").

Partner of community. All not-for-profit healthcare organizations and some for-profit healthcare organizations collaborate with their communities. As healthcare has become a bigger and bigger business, many organizations have moved away from community

Exhibit 2.5: What Community Benefits Can and Should Be Achieved?

Typical Planning Impact	Area	Desirable Planning Impact
Yes	Needed services provided	Yes
Little or none	Community health improvement	Some
Little or none	Partner of community	Some
Little or none	Population health management	Some

© 2017 Veralon Partners Inc.

partnering. Meaningfully carrying out the typical healthcare organization's mission of "effective caring" in an increasingly complex world would seem to require more and better interrelationships with the vast array of community agencies and groups that could contribute to this end. Greater sensitivity to the social determinants of health has raised the profile of community partnerships, and some health systems are delivering a more coordinated set of services that include coordination with community organizations. Other health systems have retreated primarily to doing what they can control through ownership and operation. Many health systems can improve their position and effectiveness through better community partnerships.

Population health management. The creation of accountable care organizations, and the emphasis on value-and-risk-based payment have ushered in the era of population health management. In its simplest form, this is the notion of taking responsibility, both clinical and financial, for the care of a defined group of people. In more evolved forms of population health management, demonstrable community health status improvement (for some or all of a defined community) is an important goal and a key success metric. Most healthcare organizations are putting the building blocks in place to manage population health; becoming competent and eventually expert in this area is an appropriately critical strategy focus for many.

Case Example: Hunterdon Healthcare Pioneers Wellness Care

Hunterdon Healthcare has been a leader in community-focused healthcare since its inception in 1953. From the outset, this medium-sized community hospital in a historically rural (but now suburban) part of New Jersey drew national attention for its emphasis on wellness and primary care.

In its 2008 strategic plan, updated in 2013, Hunterdon Healthcare continued its progressive history of service to the community. Its vision—"Hunterdon Healthcare is a national model for providing community-focused healthcare that is consumer-centered and driven by a passion for clinical excellence"—is not a slogan, but a guidepost for all that Hunterdon Healthcare (2014) does. Hunterdon Healthcare believes that building a healthier community is not an innovative program, but a grassroots effort to change people's behavior. The organization pursues this goal in part by giving patients the tools needed to make healthier choices in order to improve their well-being.

For five years in a row (through 2014, the latest data available), Hunterdon County has been rated the healthiest county in New Jersey by the Robert Wood Johnson Foundation and the University of Wisconsin Population Health Institute. This outcome is, at least in part, the result of Hunterdon Healthcare's increasingly geographically distributed primary care and ambulatory care service network (more than 80 percent of local residents claim to have a primary care physician, a very high percentage). These networks are supported by a diverse array of Hunterdon Healthcare wellness services including nutrition, exercise, and other key lifestyle-related programs. The organization has had a program called Partnership for Health with more than 40 organizations in its community for more than 20 years to provide education, outreach resources, and programs that contribute to better prevention and, ultimately, better health. While many other organizations are just beginning to focus on population health, Hunterdon Healthcare has been a leader in this for many years.

Going forward, Hunterdon Healthcare's strategy is to be an invaluable healthcare resource for the communities it serves, an approach that entails three key pillars: providing the best value, improving health, and simplifying healthcare. Being a "resource" means continuing to go above and beyond its role as a provider of healthcare services and truly contributing in a broad and meaningful way to population health.

CONCLUSION

Strategic planning must become more outcome oriented. Good process is important, and will remain so, but tangible benefits, not just a feel-good ending, need to be achieved. Deriving benefits starts, at the outset of the process, with identifying and communicating categories and types of benefits that could be realized through strategic planning.

This chapter has reviewed four different types of substantive benefit (product or market, financial, operational, community) and 16 subcategories of possible benefits in these broad categories. Leadership needs to agree on which benefits should be realized through the strategic planning effort, and the process needs to keep these potential benefits highly visible and to continually drive toward their realization. An orientation toward benefits realization will make future strategic planning more relevant and effective and help lead strategic planning into a new era of prominence as an important discipline in healthcare organizations.

REFERENCES

Hunterdon Healthcare. 2014. *2014 Report to the Community*. Accessed November 30, 2016. www.hunterdonhealthcare.org/wp-content/uploads/2015/02/HH_Report-to-the-Community_2014.pdf.

Institute of Medicine. 1999. *To Err Is Human: Building a Safer Health System*. Washington, DC: National Academies Press.

Setting the Stage
for Successful
Strategic Planning

CHAPTER 3

Organizing for Success

There is in that act of preparation the moment
you start caring.

—*Winston Churchill*

The only difference between a mob and a
trained army is organization.

—*Calvin Coolidge*

Thoughtful and purposeful preparation is critical before beginning
the actual work of strategic planning. Without the right prep work,
even the most well-designed planning process with objectively sound
outputs can fall flat. The following chapter discusses 12 steps, rep-
resenting four key categories of preparation, that leadership teams
should complete in advance of strategic planning to minimize avoidable challenges and maximize the chances of planning and plan
success.

COMMUNICATION AND EXPECTATIONS

The concept of communication is integral to the first six steps of
organizing for strategic planning; however, it remains critical to
success throughout planning and especially during the transition

to implementation. To ensure a high level of organizational participation and engagement, emphasize communication of strategic planning objectives, as well as the proposed planning process, and schedule from the outset.

Step 1: Identify and Communicate Desired Strategic Planning Outcomes

The importance of clear outcomes to successful strategic planning cannot be overstated. Outcomes-oriented statements such as "strategic planning will provide our organization with a road map for the future" or "strategic planning will allow our organization to allocate scarce resources in the most effective manner possible" are too general to warrant the time, resources, and focus that strategic planning requires.

In addition, proactively setting clear primary objectives promotes staying on track after planning begins. Objectives should be clear signposts that are periodically revisited as planning takes shape to demonstrate progress and encourage a sustained focus on the issues that matter most. Desired objectives for the modern healthcare strategic planning process may include determining how to

- coordinate and integrate care across the care continuum;
- increase access to services, especially primary and other ambulatory care services;
- effectively align hospitals and physicians to manage the health of populations;
- respond to increased consumerism, including demands for more person-centric care delivery and transparency of information;
- prepare for and respond to provider and payer market consolidation; and
- achieve the best clinical outcomes at the lowest cost.

Step 2: Describe and Communicate the Planning Process

Too often, planning begins without an understanding of what the planning process entails. Without a clear sense of the sequencing of activities and the ideal progression, planning participants will have varied expectations of what is to be done and in what order; this situation may result in key stakeholders feeling reluctant to participate in the planning process or the feeling removed from it entirely. Even if key stakeholders do engage, the lack of clarity in approach may yield planning efforts that are unfocused, inefficient, and even unproductive. Worse, it can lead to broader organizational confusion and skepticism about strategic planning and the strategy it generates.

To proactively avoid these challenges, prior to initiating strategic planning it is imperative to outline a stepwise planning process that is appropriately customized to meet your organization's specific needs. Whether or not your organization chooses to follow the strategic planning process delineated in this book, teams should clearly define and document the activities for and the outputs of each step. Then this information must be communicated effectively to leadership and all other key stakeholders.

Step 3: Establish and Communicate the Strategic Planning Schedule

Although strategic planning should be an ongoing activity and not simply a punctuated event, development of a comprehensive strategic plan or a complete update of the current plan usually occurs every three years. Comprehensive plan development or updating requires a more detailed and structured time line as compared to routine updates and ongoing strategic planning activities, but both should have formally established schedules.

As with the previous two steps, and particularly for more comprehensive planning efforts, the planning team should determine the schedule of the strategic planning process before planning activities are initiated, and they should clearly communicate it to all relevant stakeholders. The schedule for comprehensive strategic plan development should align with the stages of the planning process developed per the previous step.

No universally accepted optimal duration of the full strategic planning process exists. Some believe the plan should be completed as quickly as possible to maintain a high degree of focus and to begin execution promptly. Others believe that an extended schedule allows for broader participation, more time to generate buy-in, and more advanced critical thinking. The authors of this book often employ a time line for a full planning process of approximately six months, falling somewhere between these two points on the spectrum, generally allowing for broad participation, but fully appreciating the value of focus and expediency.

MANAGEMENT AND LEADERSHIP

Step 4: Assert CEO Leadership of Strategic Planning

In nearly all organizations, including healthcare organizations, the CEO actively champions and leads the strategic planning process. Other leaders may also play important roles, and in a not-for-profit organization the board of directors is especially critical. However, the CEO should be the primary leader.

C. Davis Fogg (2010) suggests clarifying key roles and responsibilities of the CEO at the outset of the strategic planning process. Roles and responsibilities of the CEO are to

- demonstrate and continually reinforce the importance of planning in the organization;

- allocate time, money, staff support, and personal support to the planning process;
- set high standards for the planning process and results;
- encourage creativity and the search for the unlikely or not so obvious;
- lead the development of an inspired, comprehensive, and far-reaching vision for the organization;
- make, push, or affirm timely decisions;
- serve as the principal link between the planning process and important external constituencies;
- hold senior staff and others accountable for results and reward them accordingly;
- install an ongoing integrated planning process and infrastructure;
- visibly champion strategic planning; and
- encourage input from all participants and avoid dominating the discussion.

By asserting a strong presence at the start of the strategic planning process and then executing key elements of the leadership role throughout, the CEO can increase the probability of smoothly functioning processes and successful results.

Step 5: Define and Formalize the Roles and Responsibilities of Other Organizational Leaders

The Board

Strategic planning is a major responsibility of a board, particularly in many not-for-profit organizations wherein the board represents the community at large. As such, the board needs to play an especially significant role in setting and guarding the mission and values of the organization (phase 2 of the four planning phases outlined in chapter 1). The board members should also serve as key advisers to senior staff on other significant plan elements. Ultimately, it is the board that must approve or reject the strategic plan.

Who, How, and How Much

There is no right answer for every organization as to who should be involved, to what extent, and via what mechanisms. Some experts believe that the senior management team is principally responsible for planning and that other stakeholders' involvement should be limited by stakeholder group type or role played. Some believe that the best plans are developed when stakeholders from all levels of an organization have opportunities to contribute, or at least formally react. The perspective espoused in this book falls closer to the latter view, within reason and without excessively or detrimentally affecting planning efficiency. Chapter 4 discusses our perspective on this issue further.

Given that no "one best way" exists, the CEO and senior management team have to make choices about participation and roles (in conjunction with the board to the extent appropriate). Regardless of what is ultimately determined, these choices should be made and clearly communicated before the planning process begins. Modifications can be made if necessary once planning begins, but each major participant group must understand expectations regarding its participation and role at the outset of the process.

The general consensus among experts, including the authors, is that for healthcare organizations, strategic planning should actively engage aligned physician leaders in determining the organization's future direction and priorities. Depending on the nature of the organization, it may be important for other clinicians to also play a key role in strategic planning. Again, which specific physician leaders and other physician representatives and in what capacities are to be determined by executive leadership.

Oversight Bodies

A strategic planning steering committee is typically established to oversee the planning process. This group typically comprises senior leadership, including physician leaders, and key board members. At the outset of the process, the steering committee should aim to accomplish the following, though the group's role becomes more expansive once planning begins:

- Develop, affirm, and set a plan to communicate the desired strategic planning outcomes.
- Affirm (or revise as necessary) the proposed strategic planning approach and time line, including identification of key milestones.
- Identify meaningful gaps in knowledge or information (internal or related to the market), peers, and sector, and propose a plan to close any gaps.
- Identify internal and external stakeholders to be interviewed.
- Identify the need for external advisers and procure this support as necessary.
- Select planning facilitation and management leads and their roles, including the strategic planning facilitator (internal or external), and all types of logistical support, including scheduling, outreach, and coordination with involved stakeholders.

Step 6: Identify the Strategic Planning Facilitator

While the CEO is the strategic planning leader, another individual typically manages day-to-day facilitation of the process. The team must resolve who will assume this responsibility and how facilitation will be carried out at the outset of the process. Once the selection is made and facilitation duties are delineated, this information should be communicated widely before strategic planning formally commences.

Fogg (2010, 31) suggests that "most CEOs depend upon a skilled, objective strategic planning facilitator to jump-start the organization into strategic planning and to shepherd the process during the early years of implementation. A good facilitator helps the organization design and install an effective planning and review process, trains the planning team and the organization in facilitation techniques, intervenes when key organizational or strategic blockages occur, and exits once the team is self-sustaining and self-facilitating." Nearly all healthcare provider organizations must choose between an internal leader, typically the director or vice president of planning, and an outside consultant for this role. In small healthcare provider organizations, the CEO or another C-suite representative may act as the strategic planning facilitator, though it can be difficult for the CEO to effectively encourage open discussion given his organizational position (see chapter 4).

CONTEXT

Step 7: Conduct Strategic Planning Orientation Meetings

Orientation meetings set the stage for the official launch of the planning process. Although meetings may be deferred until the strategic planning process formally commences, these meetings should be scheduled during the preplanning stage.

To become fully engaged at the outset of the process and to provide important context as backdrop for the plan, senior management and the strategic planning steering committee might embark on a planning retreat. Here leadership and other committee members explore important environmental trends and their potential implications and preliminarily identify key strategic issues for the organization. As described in more detail in the next section, such a planning retreat often also serves as a forum to review the organization's past planning initiatives, including successes and failures.

Holding strategic planning orientation sessions for other groups in the organization may be desirable at this point as well. Depending on the size and complexity of the organization and the breadth and depth of participation being sought in the strategic planning process, orientation sessions may be held with the entire board, other members of senior management, physicians, other professional staff, key external community leaders, or some combination of these. These sessions usually focus on a few of the areas outlined, such as objectives for strategic planning, the planning process and time line, or the role of the affected constituencies in the planning process.

Step 8: Review Past Strategies and Identify Successes and Failures

A review of the organization's past strategies, successes, and failures is often best completed before the strategic planning process formally starts.

An objective review of past strategies can be enlightening. Often the actual strategies an organization used were different from those proposed in the strategic plan. Similarly, the actual strategies the organization employed may vary from those that leadership thought were being followed. A review of historical documents by someone outside the inner circle—a new senior staff member or a consultant—and a discussion of what was proposed, what was perceived, and what actually occurred over the previous three to five years can be a fascinating and important pre–planning process exercise. This review can also help identify shortcomings in the past process for implementing strategies and tracking results, thereby building support for better implementation approaches in the proposed planning effort.

As part of this process, the team should review what has worked, what has not, and why. Failure to pay adequate attention to unsuccessful strategies in formal planning can lead to recurring mistakes.

Step 9: Assemble Relevant Historical Data

Possessing accurate and relevant data is an asset to strategic planning. Conversely, having inaccurate and incomplete data, or the inability to assemble a comprehensive set of data, can be a major impediment to strategic planning. As such, it is never too early to begin assembling key data to support the environmental assessment phase of planning. Chapter 6 discusses the specific types of data required for successful strategic planning and analytical approaches. Generally, relevant historical data should profile the past three or so years of the organization's performance and position and the market in which it operates.

To get an early start on the time-consuming data collection process, organizations must be proactive in the identification and aggregation of necessary data. Further, taking a proactive stance is a critical element of a good data collection and organization time line. Discovering at the middle or end of the process that essential data are missing or inaccurate is discouraging at a minimum and disabling at worst, especially if the problem is discovered in a public forum and undermines the credibility of the strategic planning process.

MIND-SET

Step 10: Resolve Not to Overanalyze Historical Data

Historical data assembled to aid strategic planning can be a great asset, but data analysis can also trap the organization in a cycle of ineffectiveness and cause excessive delays. Planning teams should avoid analyzing every facet of historical performance or a few participants' overestimation of the impact that more, or more detailed, data will have on future strategy. Both challenges can derail the planning process and inappropriately bring into question the validity of data or analytic methods—they should be proactively mitigated.

In order to avoid wasteful and distracting overanalysis, the strategic planning facilitator and the CEO should make decisions about the data to be examined and the analytic methods used, in consultation with other senior leaders as appropriate, and communicate to all planning participants. In addition, the planning facilitator must consistently reinforce the notion that while historical data may help to define the problem, they are not the only—or even the most important—factor in determining key challenges, and they certainly are not the answer.

Although focusing on the past and dwelling on the familiar can be comforting, strategic planning should be oriented toward the future. Organizations should resolve to use historical data for their intended purposes as defined, communicated, and reiterated by the planning facilitator and steering committee leaders.

Step 11: Prepare to Stimulate New Thinking

Meaningful Strategic Planning

As the strategic planning process gets under way, teams must resist the temptation to extrapolate from past performance and experience to devise future strategy. In the more orderly and less frenetic world of past decades, passable and even good strategic planning may have resulted from this approach. But with nonlinear and fast-paced changes in the field, extrapolation would now likely lead to naive strategies at best and incorrect forecasts and flawed strategic direction at worst. Moreover, as highlighted in chapter 1, organizations must overcome the urge to focus primarily on operational effectiveness—doing the same things competitors do but more efficiently or with more favorable results—and engage in planning that yields more sustainable and meaningful competitive advantages.

Avoiding Mimicry

Another problematic strategic planning method healthcare organizations frequently use is adopting or mimicking strategies used by other organizations in demographically similar but more advanced regional markets. This practice is most often seen when organizations in less advanced markets try to replicate a successful strategy implemented in California, Massachusetts, or a similarly advanced market. Although this approach may be appealing and may ultimately do no harm, it poses significant hazards, including the failure to truly understand one's market and develop strategies and plans that address more pertinent local market needs.

While potentially positive learning can occur in these situations, teams should emphasize creating a plan that effectively creates competitive advantages suited to an organization's strengths, opportunities, and unique market. As described in chapters 6, 7, and 8, healthcare planners must be thoughtful and intuitive in their characterization of the future environment, understanding implications of changing environmental conditions and considering strategies that might not make a large difference today but will be of potential critical importance tomorrow. Unfortunately, much strategic planning conducted by healthcare organizations assumes a static competitive environment, or at least underestimates the degree and pace of change that will occur. Such a mind-set is even more dangerous than inappropriate mimicry given how dynamic the field has been in recent years (and will likely be in the future).

Promoting Creative Thinking

Preparation for the strategic planning process in each organization should include some review and summary of the enormous body of available strategic thinking literature, the incorporation of planning exercises designed to contemplate alternatives that may seem radical today, and the use of planning techniques that may help the organization leap, rather than step, forward in its strategic development (see chapters 5 and 12 for more information on innovative thinking).

Step 12: Reinforce a Future Orientation

To successfully plan for the future, healthcare organizations must adopt a new perspective. This perspective must be broader, bolder, and more creative and dynamic than any required in the past. To counter the tendency to overemphasize past and present circumstances, leaders need to overcompensate actively and continually push their organizations to break with that past and consider alternative futures that differ vastly from what they know today. Injecting this kind of thinking into healthcare strategic planning invigorates the process and leads to thoughtful plans and strategies that will set the new standard by which successful planning and strategy development are measured in the twenty-first century.

CONCLUSION

Even 30 years after its emergence, healthcare strategic planning remains a relatively immature practice, though there is evidence of growing sophistication. In this chapter alone, healthcare strategic planning has been characterized as historically focused rather than future oriented, lacking creativity, preoccupied with mimicry, haphazardly applied, and poorly prepared for. One part of the problem is a lack of drive toward clear, compelling results; another is inadequate planning preparation by leaders, staff, and other key stakeholders. This chapter addresses both of these potential deficits and, it is hoped, heightens awareness of the need to prepare for successful strategic planning.

REFERENCE

Fogg, C. D. 2010. *Team-Based Strategic Planning: A Complete Guide to Structuring, Facilitating, and Implementing the Process.* N. p.: CreateSpace Independent Publishing Platform.

CHAPTER 4

Major Planning Process Considerations

It is good to have an end to journey toward; but it is the journey that matters, in the end.

—Ursula K. LeGuin

The most important things a leader can bring to a changing organization are passion, conviction, and confidence in others. Too often executives announce a plan, launch a task force, and then simply hope that people find the answers— instead of offering a dream, stretching their horizons, and encouraging people to do the same. That is why we say, "Leaders go first . . ."

—Rosabeth Moss Kanter

Structuring and carrying out an effective strategic planning process is often more important to a healthcare organization, and to the success of strategic planning, than the plan itself. The increasing complexity of the healthcare environment and growing vulnerability of provider organizations to myriad external threats have made it far more challenging to effectively carry out strategic planning and develop strategy.

At the same time, the increasing size, diversity, and complexity of healthcare organizations make for unwieldy entities to communicate in and to manage. While it is possible to overdo the strategic planning process and derail or overwhelm the organization's capacities, in general more process is better than less. As a rule, organizations should strive to maximize participation in the planning process within the limits of their capabilities to handle it and achieve the desired results.

The key to an effective planning process is developing shared understanding—and ultimately consensus—about four important elements of the strategic plan:

- Current, and especially future, environment
- Critical issues the organization faces
- Mission and vision to guide the organization to the future
- Major plan outputs, including priority strategies and alternatives considered

An effective process builds acceptance, facilitates approval, and expedites the transition from planning to action.

The planning process needs to link effectively the many constituencies involved in healthcare organizations. If it does, it can facilitate better communication among staff and improved coherence in future operations. While the organization should certainly seek tangible outputs from strategic planning, the planning process presents important opportunities for improving communication across the organization and for forging new and stronger bonds among stakeholder individuals and groups to help ensure the organization's future viability.

This chapter addresses some of the critical elements of the planning process. While many of these elements have been mentioned in passing in previous chapters, the importance of a strong planning process calls for more extended discussion.

FACILITATION

Facilitation is an extremely critical element of a successful strategic planning process. Someone needs to be primarily responsible for guiding the process throughout, ensuring that the important planning tasks are conducted and completed, assisting leadership and other key groups involved in the process in reaching decisions and achieving consensus, and then directing the transition from planning to successful implementation. While many individuals involved in the strategic planning process will have specific responsibility for facilitating one or two aspects of the diverse group work, one person typically takes the lead throughout, with overriding responsibilities for the entire process.

What alternatives exist for effective facilitation of the strategic planning process? Many healthcare organizations have a planning staff or organizational development department (or occasionally other internal resources) that can facilitate the planning process. Some organizations retain consultants to fill this role. When evaluating possible consultants, organizations should look for individuals who are highly experienced, have healthcare field and comparable organization experience, and possess a range of facilitation skills described further in the following sections.

In some instances, the CEO may consider serving as the process facilitator. Most CEOs find this job extremely challenging, if for no other reason than it makes productive group discussion and consensus development difficult. Most CEOs inhibit free discussion as a result of their power and authority and tend to dominate meetings when put in charge. Avoid this alternative if at all possible.

C. Davis Fogg (2010) suggests that the best facilitators have three types of skills (see exhibit 4.1):

- Process: putting the planning process together and making it work
- Content: giving specific solutions to business and strategic problems
- Intervention: breaking personal, organization, and business decision blockages

He adds that all three types of skills may not be, and often are not, possessed by any single individual. The more of the three skills

Exhibit 4.1: The Facilitator's Job Description

What the Facilitator Does

I. PROCESS

- Structure
  - Structures the process
  - Defines key analyses
  - Produces the manual
  - Handles documentation
- Training
  - Trains in planning and process
- Facilitation
  - Facilitates major meetings
  - Teaches others to facilitate
  - Gives private advice on process
  - Schedules meetings
- Resourcing
  - Identifies training
  - Identifies outside facilitators
  - Identifies content specialists

II. CONTENT

- Solutions to specific strategic issues

III. INTERVENTION

- Diagnostic interviewing
  - Initial
  - In process
- Private counsel, particularly CEO
- Team interventions
- Keeps process on time

What the Facilitator Does Not Do

- Develop the plan
- Write the plan
- Make decisions
- Become a power point
- Play politics
- Execute the plan

When the Boss Facilitates; Is Part of the Team

- Be a member of the group
- Speak last
- Use good facilitator skills
- Be neutral
- Let the team come to consensus
- Do not dominate or be authoritarian
- You always have the deciding vote—use it sparingly

Source: Fogg (2010). Used with permission.

that are offered by one person or group, the more effective and efficient the strategic planning process will be. In nearly every strategic planning effort, the organization needs all three types of skills, and it must be prepared to provide them at appropriate points in the process. Fogg believes that the lead facilitator must have certain basic process skills, especially a keen understanding of all parts of the planning and implementation process, and must know how to weave them together successfully. She must also have knowledge of organizational behavior and the change process and strong leadership capabilities.

TEAMWORK

Much of the strategic planning process occurs through the efforts of informally or formally constituted, diverse groups. In the typical strategic planning process, important team work is performed by the strategic planning committee, board of trustees, senior management staff, and a variety of standing or ad hoc groups. How can the effectiveness of these many and varied groups be maximized?

Fogg (2010, 257) suggests that effective teams are "characterized by:

- Considerable discussion
- Open communication
- Debate, even conflict, on key issues
- Decision by consensus whenever possible
- Monitoring, measuring, and correcting of their own team behaviors"

Effective teams must also have a clear charge or objective to accomplish, good leadership by a chair who facilitates and directs but does not dominate, and accountability of the team and individual members for results. Among other qualities, individual team members must be good listeners, constructive participants, and willing to put aside their own self-interest for the sake of the group. All in all, a very tall order, but one that is essential to the smooth and successful flow of activities in the strategic planning process.

The interaction of the facilitator and team is a critical element of an effective strategic planning process. Fogg (2010) provides an extremely useful checklist (see exhibit 4.2) of facilitation tips to keep the teams on track and moving ahead.

Exhibit 4.2: Team Interventions

Process
- Facilitate team mission; roles, job description, and processes used
- Process checks during and at end of meetings—what is good and bad versus norms
- Redirect process when off track
- Point out dysfunctional team behavior

Meeting
- Off agenda/subject—get team back on track
- Summarize/crystallize key points; transitions
- Offer stand-up facilitation when team is bogged down
- Crystallize/facilitate/resolve conflicts
- Missing the point—suggest it

Content
- Wrong decision—point out correct options/process to define correct decision
- Suggest expert outsiders
- Give specific content solutions

Individual
- Point out dysfunctional individual behavior or interactions
- Offer individual/pair counseling

Source: Fogg (2010).

PLANNING RETREATS

Almost every strategic planning process has at least one planning retreat. The retreat usually brings together board members, physicians, and other clinicians and members of management in an extended planning session. Some retreats are intended for board members exclusively, while others are for members of different leadership groups. Depending on the organization's style and preferences, as well as the particular focus of the retreat, the retreat may be held off-site and may even be carried out in a remote location combined with social and recreational activities. The following section presents a review of the purposes of the different types of retreats that may be held.

Kickoff Retreat

Some organizations use a retreat at the beginning of strategic planning to jump-start the process and create enthusiasm and momentum. The agenda for this type of retreat may include some or all of the following:

- Rationale for strategic planning (purpose, expected benefits)
- Strategic planning orientation (see chapter 3)
- Review of previous planning efforts, successes, and failures
- Review of the organization's recent performance
- Discussion of the organization's strengths, weaknesses, opportunities, and threats
- Review of current major strategic initiatives
- Identification on a preliminary basis of major planning issues

Often, one or more outside keynote speakers are used to discuss critical issues or environmental challenges. If external speakers present, they should be oriented to the organization's situation and their content previewed with the facilitator to ensure it is on topic and avoids statements that distract rather than enlighten. This type of retreat is a good vehicle for underscoring the importance of strategic planning and creating heightened interest in the planning process from the outset.

Midprocess Retreat

At any number of points in the middle of the strategic planning process, retreats can be held to do the following:

- Focus on a particular issue of concern
- Have extended discussion that is not possible in a regular planning committee session
- Obtain broad-based input, including input from the members of the planning committee and other important leaders not represented on the committee
- Brainstorm about approaches to issues facing the organization

External speakers may be used in midprocess retreats in a manner similar to kickoff retreats. The purposes of the midprocess retreat are information sharing, clarification, and direction. Sometimes this retreat is referred to as the "question" retreat—the attendees make sure the organization is focusing on the right strategic questions. These retreats are rarely used for decision making or communicating "answers" to strategic planning issues.

Concluding Retreat

At or near the end of the strategic planning process, a retreat may be held to

- obtain additional, broad-based input before finalizing the recommendations;
- communicate the answers (i.e., the plan's key recommendations);
- serve as a bridge to implementation, including strategizing about implementation opportunities and barriers; and
- build a broader consensus on the plan and its recommendations than that offered by the planning committee alone.

Often, this type of retreat is developed to expose all members of the board to a plan before it is brought to this group for formal consideration of its adoption. This type of retreat may also be used to signal to the organization that planning is (temporarily) over and implementation is about to begin.

Retreats may also be held in off years, when the organization is not undertaking a full strategic planning effort, to accomplish any of the purposes cited earlier and to keep the planning process going even as the organization's efforts are primarily devoted to implementation. Increasingly, healthcare organizations are using one or two planning retreats per year to review and revise the strategic plan, make important corrections to the direction and strategies, and obtain broad-based consensus on key initiatives to keep the organization moving forward. (See chapter 10 for more discussion of the annual strategic plan update and the potential role of retreats.) These retreats are an excellent vehicle for maintaining momentum and organizational commitment in the face of constant day-to-day pressures that consume management and have the potential to take the organization off course.

RESEARCH APPROACHES

Much of the success of the strategic planning process is dependent on information gathering and the involvement of key constituencies, which comes through various research efforts. The importance of constructive involvement of key constituencies in the strategic planning process cannot be overstated; implementation is dependent on a broad base of support for the plan's recommendations and actions. This support is only likely to occur if stakeholders believe they have a true opportunity to shape the results. A brief review of the range of research approaches used in strategic planning follows.

Interviews

Interviewing is typically part of every strategic planning process. Individual or group interviews usually occur early in the strategic planning process to gather information and demonstrate sensitivity to the perspectives of internal parties, and they are also intended to accomplish one or both of these purposes with external parties. Sometimes, interviews may be carried out during the middle of the process to gather additional information on issues of concern or involve select parties in review of alternative approaches for addressing particular issues.

Surveys

Surveys are the second most frequently employed technique, and are often used for information gathering early in the strategic planning process. Many organizations participate in ongoing survey efforts that provide valuable input for strategic planning—patient satisfaction, quality and outcomes tracking, and consumer perception are among the most common. Surveys may be carried out internally to gather broad input in a less expensive way than possible through other research approaches. Internal surveys may also allow each member of an affected group to be involved in the strategic planning process and to accomplish this participation in an equitable and consistent manner. External surveys have similar purposes. The advantages and disadvantages of different survey approaches—electronic, mail, or telephone—as information-gathering techniques are best left to experts in this subject area (e.g., *Designing and Conducting Survey Research: A Comprehensive Guide* by Louis M. Rea and Richard A. Parker). With the availability and prevalence of electronic communication today and the rise of various standard online survey tools, much focused surveying occurs at a relatively low cost via the Internet or organizational intranets.

Focus Groups

The focus group technique is the least frequently used of the three approaches, but it is growing more commonplace in strategic planning processes. Focus groups may be convened at any point in the process to gather information on a particular issue. Such groups are becoming more widely used in the strategy formulation stage of the planning process and provide excellent forums for multidisciplinary development of strategy on a given issue. The advantages and disadvantages of focus groups versus other research approaches is a larger subject than can be addressed here (e.g., *Focus Groups: A Practical Guide for Applied Research* by Richard A. Krueger and Mary Anne Casey).

Reactor Panels

The reactor panel is a modified version of the focus group. Depending on the substance of the material to which a reaction is being sought, reactor panel members may be key constituents of a particular group (e.g., cardiovascular providers) or more diverse in representation (e.g., the medical executive committee). When conducting a reactor panel during the strategic planning process, the facilitator is usually seeking a found response to a particular recommendation, set of recommendations, or potential alterations under consideration. Reactor panels are appropriate vehicles for these narrowly defined purposes.

Most strategic planning processes employ more than one of these approaches. With the growing recognition of the importance of a strong process in strategic planning, organizations will likely pursue more extensive use of individual and group research approaches in future strategic planning efforts.

KEY STAKEHOLDER INVOLVEMENT

The strategic planning process is more likely to succeed if all key stakeholders understand their roles. The following sections briefly describe each major group's role.

Board Members

The strategic planning committee is usually an ad hoc or standing committee of the board and therefore includes significant representation from the board of directors. Board members are important participants in retreats, and they are involved in internal research. The board should be concerned with the policy implications of strategic planning and is generally and appropriately focused on the organizational direction portion of the strategic planning output.

Physicians

In hospitals, health systems, and, obviously, medical groups, physicians should be well represented on the strategic planning committee. They are often solicited for input, and, moreover, they often provide the most extensive contributions of all internal (and sometimes external) constituencies.

Physicians concern themselves with the clinical implications of strategic planning; in teaching hospitals and academic medical centers, they are also interested in teaching and research interrelationships with clinical services and specific recommendations affecting the academic role of their organizations. Physicians may be most broadly affected by the outputs of the strategic planning process; however, excepting some of the second- or later-generation integrated delivery systems, they do not have direct approval authority or clear implementation responsibility.

Few topics are as hotly debated today as how to involve medical staff members in hospital and health system strategic planning. The escalation of competition between physicians and hospitals over provision of outpatient services and, increasingly, entire high-margin clinical service lines, has created enormous complexity and confusion in this area. In addition, some physician groups are bearing risk for the total cost of patient care, sometimes leading them to view the hospital, with its typically higher-cost services, as the enemy. However, with more physicians employed by hospitals and health systems, this dynamic has begun changing in recent years. These alignments and competitive postures yield an ever-evolving mix of tension and cooperation between a hospital and its medical staff that must be considered in its uniqueness in each market.

While no single approach exists that fits every situation, constructive and careful physician involvement in the planning process is vital to effective planning. Organizations need to make appropriate accommodations for competitive considerations in many instances. Little or no involvement of physicians in strategic planning is not an option.

Senior Management

Senior management is almost always represented on the strategic planning committee, but it is generally fewer in number and lesser in "voice" than board members or physicians. Management, however, plays an important and central role as the coordinator of the strategic planning process—structuring, staffing, keeping it moving along, and overseeing implementation. Senior management's roles and responsibilities in the process generally increase as the planning reaches its later stages.

Other Clinicians

Depending on the nature of the organization, other clinicians (e.g., nurses, physical therapists, psychologists) may play a major or minor role in the strategic planning process. In healthcare organizations not dominated by hospitals or physicians, other clinicians may have significant involvement, including participation on the strategic planning committee of the board. In hospital- or physician-dominated healthcare organizations, other clinicians play a minimal role in the strategic planning process, but they usually get involved when implementation begins or is near.

Other Management

In most cases, other management members only get involved in the strategic planning process prior to implementation if a significant issue or area of concern arises over which they have direct responsibility or expertise.

Although some strategic planning experts advocate a bottom-up strategic planning process that calls for broad-based and extensive participation from all levels of the organization, few healthcare organizations practice such an approach (more about this situation follows later in the chapter). A summary of the typical involvement of key stakeholder groups in major elements of the planning process appears as exhibit 4.3. While every planning process is carried out somewhat differently, exhibit 4.3 summarizes the information in the previous sections and can be used as an initial framework for structuring involvement at the outset of strategic planning. It may be reconsidered as the process moves along.

ADVANCING TO THE NEXT LEVEL: BOTTOM-UP VERSUS TOP-DOWN STRATEGIC PLANNING

Strategic planning in healthcare is still very much a top-down process. Dominated by senior management (see exhibit 4.4), and to some degree, the board, planning in most organizations engenders little participation, awareness, and ultimately support from the majority of employees, and even less from customers. Strategic planning in large healthcare organizations is still very hierarchical, with business units and other subsidiary entities reacting and responding to edicts and directives from on high.

Practices in leading organizations outside of healthcare are almost exactly the opposite. While corporate leadership provides high-level direction and guidance, planning is increasingly focused in the business units or other subsidiary parts of the company and driven up, rather than down, through the organization.

A bottom-up approach has many benefits: It allows broader-based, more substantial, and more meaningful participation in the planning process; generally encourages creativity and innovation;

Select Process Elements

Select Groups/Individuals	Approval	Steering Committee	Interviews/ Surveys	Retreat	Strategy Formulation	Implementation
Entire board	✓			✓		Oversight
Planning committee of the board	✓	✓	✓	✓	✓	Direction and management
Other leadership and management		✓	✓	✓	✓	✓
Physicians			✓	✓	✓	✓
Staff			✓			✓
Community			✓			
Planning staff	←——————————— Support entire process ———————————→					

© 2017 Veralon Partners Inc.

Exhibit 4.4: Participation of Stakeholders in Healthcare Strategic Planning

	1 No Participation	2 Limited Participation	3 Moderate Participation	4 Considerable Participation	5 Extensive Participation	N/A Unsure	Mean Response
Board members	5% (20)	20% (78)	27% (103)	26% (101)	18% (69)	3% (13)	3.33
Physicians	3% (12)	19% (72)	35% (133)	30% (113)	12% (46)	1% (5)	3.29
Other clinicians	9% (35)	35% (131)	33% (124)	17% (63)	4% (14)	2% (9)	2.70
Senior management	0% (1)	2% (9)	7% (26)	26% (99)	64% (247)	0% (1)	4.52
Middle management	5% (19)	21% (82)	38% (146)	29% (111)	6% (22)	1% (3)	3.09
Outside community leaders	31% (119)	39% (148)	18% (70)	8% (30)	1% (5)	3% (10)	2.07
Outside customers/ patients	38% (147)	39% (149)	14% (55)	4% (15)	1% (3)	3% (13)	1.86
					Total Respondents		384

has the "real action" of planning taking place closer to the customer; facilitates organizational support for what results from the planning process; and leads to greater implementation success. In addition to senior management providing vision and direction and championing the process, such organizations must have a culture of trust and accountability, outstanding formal and informal communication networks, and sound strategic skills across the organization.

A decentralized planning process is much harder to manage than a centralized one, and, of course, such a process risks loss of control. However, leading companies have found that the benefits of a decentralized process far outweigh the negatives and that it delivers much more overall value. Some organizations are beginning to move in this direction, but as a field, much progress is needed to approach this best practice inside of healthcare.

EVOLVING AND IMPROVING THE PROCESS

Even today, too many healthcare organizations are wedded to a process that has worked well historically and are reluctant to make significant changes. Some ask, why fix what isn't broken? While there is value and security in the tried and true, regular advances in approaches and methods are occurring in strategic planning in healthcare (and outside of it). Therefore, aspects of a process that is five or ten years old—or even one year—may not be current enough to keep the organization in the forefront. Executives certainly aren't content with yesterday's operations management or financial planning and management approaches, so why shouldn't planning evolve too?

The quality and continuous improvement orientation of an organization's strategic planning process can be evaluated by examining the process at three increasingly challenging levels of inquiry:

1. Is the current process comprehensive, objective, timely, and highly participatory throughout the organization? This question is the most basic.
2. Does the process link effectively to operations and to individual and group performance objectives in the organization?
3. Does the process include continuous learning so that process deficiencies are identified and corrected before the next planning cycle begins?

Organizations with flexible, continuously improving planning processes are able to adapt more readily to the changing environment that is characteristic of healthcare today. These organizations employ planning processes that are far more externally oriented than the typical healthcare organization. They use external factors and forces to create the platform for change that is necessary to keep strategic planning alive and vital.

CONCLUSION

This chapter illustrates that the impact of an effective strategic planning process is at least as important to organizational success as the actual plan itself. When structured and carried out with care, the facilitation, planning retreats, research, and involvement of key stakeholders can lead to a highly successful planning process that maximizes participation and secures a commitment to plan implementation.

SUGGESTED READINGS

Krueger, R. A., and M. A. Casey. 2015. *Focus Groups: A Practical Guide for Applied Research*, 5th ed. Thousand Oaks, CA: Sage Publications, Inc.

Rea, L. M., and R. A. Parker. 2014. *Designing and Conducting Survey Research: A Comprehensive Guide*, 4th ed. San Francisco: Jossey-Bass.

REFERENCE

Fogg, C. D. 2010. *Team-Based Strategic Planning: A Complete Guide to Structuring, Facilitating, and Implementing the Process.* N. p.: CreateSpace Independent Publishing Platform.

Encouraging Strategic Thinking

I insist on a lot of time being spent, almost every day,
to just sit and think.

—*Warren Buffett*

Leadership is not just about doing things, it is also about
thinking. Make time for it.

—*Freek Vermeulen*

WHAT IS STRATEGIC THINKING?

This question is puzzling to most, if not all, healthcare executives and even strategic planning professionals. This question has been addressed most frequently and successfully outside the context of healthcare, but the hypotheses and definitions proposed in response are nonetheless relevant to healthcare executives. Chapter 5 presents a review of writings on the topic, much of them from the late twentieth century, when the roles of strategic planning and strategic thinking were hotly debated. These early insights may be useful for healthcare leaders seeking to clarify—or refresh—their approach to the topic.

Henry Mintzberg (1994, 107), in his landmark devastating critique of strategic planning, says, "Strategic planning isn't strategic thinking. One is analysis and the other is synthesis . . . [strategic thinking] involves intuition and creativity. The outcome of strategic thinking is an integrated perspective of the enterprise, a not-too-precisely articulated vision of direction."

Bob Garratt (1995, 8) argues that

> strategic thinking is essentially a process . . . to see, hear and use ingeniously the . . . signals which can give competitive advantage. . . . It requires the ability to create a "holistic" view of the interconnections between apparently contradictory trends in [the] environment . . . and reframe the current mindsets which you and your competitors hold.

Garratt (1995, 2) further asserts that "'strategic thinking' is the process by which an organization's direction-givers can rise above the daily managerial processes and crises to gain different perspectives of the internal and external dynamics causing change in their environment and thereby give more effective direction to their organization."

Other writers have also contributed to the thinking on the topic. Michael E. Porter (1987, 18) notes that "strategic thinking rarely occurs spontaneously. Without formal planning systems, day-to-day concerns prevail. The future is forgotten. Formal planning provides the discipline to pause occasionally to think about strategic issues." P. Hanford (1995) adds that "'strategic thinking' in essence amounts to a richer and more creative way of thinking about and managing key issues and opportunities facing your organization. . . . Strategic thinking underscores both the formulation and implementation of your organization's effective strategy" (see exhibit 5.1).

While executives and board members may have a thorough understanding of and strong skills in operational thinking, Hanford argues that the needs are great for strong strategic thinking skills (see exhibit 5.2), and far less has been done to develop these skills.

Richard Rumelt (2011, 2) comments that "the core of strategy work is always the same: discovering the critical factors in a situation and designing a way of coordinating and focusing actions to

Exhibit 5.1: Purposes of Strategic Thinking

In the setting of direction	"Locating, attracting, and holding customers is the purpose of strategic thinking" (Hickman and Silva 1984).
In establishing "the change agenda"	"Most organizations are effective in many of the things they do and deliver. Strategic thinking is about identifying what to change, modify, add, delete or acquire" (Kaufman 1991).
In resource allocation	"Strategic thinking is about making the best use of what will always be a limited amount and quality of resources" (Hanford 1983).

Source: Garratt (1995). Reproduced with permission of The McGraw-Hill Companies.

Exhibit 5.2: Distinguishing Between Strategic and Operational Thinking

Strategic Thinking	Operational Thinking
• Longer term	• Immediate term
• Conceptual	• Concrete
• Reflective or learning	• Action or doing
• Identification of key issues and opportunities	• Resolution of existing performance problems
• Breaking new ground	• Routine and ongoing
• Effectiveness	• Efficiency
• "Hands off" approach	• "Hands on" approach
• "Helicopter" perspective	• "On the ground" perspective

Source: Hanford (1995) in Garratt (1995). Reproduced with permission of The McGraw-Hill Companies.

deal with those factors. A leader's most important responsibility is identifying the biggest challenges to forward progress and devising a coherent approach to overcoming them." Or, as Peter M. Ginter, W. Jack Duncan, and Linda E. Swayne (2013, 16) say it, "Strategic thinkers are always questioning: What are we doing now that we should stop doing? What are we not doing now, but should start doing? What are we doing now that we should continue to do but perhaps in a fundamentally different way?"

Mintzberg's thoughts have application here as well. He concludes that if strategic planning is to become truly effective and provoke serious organizational change, it needs to move beyond "preservation and rearrangement of established categories . . . and invent new ones. . . . Formal planning has promoted strategies that are extrapolated from the past or copied from others. . . . Strategy making needs to function beyond the boxes, to encourage the informal learning that produces new perspectives and new combinations" (Mintzberg 1994, 109).

How does an organization break out of the box and insert creativity, intuition, a future orientation, new perspectives, and new categories into its process for and results of strategic planning? How can strategic planning better rise to Mintzberg's challenge and be a catalyst for critical organizational change?

STRATEGIC THINKING VERSUS STRATEGIC PLANNING

Michel Robert (1998, 30) remarks that "the strategic thinking process . . . can be described as the type of thinking that attempts to determine what an organization should look like in the future." Strategic planning, historically, has been primarily concerned with how to get there; operations is all about "how." Robert (1998, 30) comments further: "Strategic thinking . . . identifies the key factors that dictate the direction of an organization, and it is a process that the organization's management uses to set direction and articulate their vision."

Robert believes there are four types of companies, as represented by the matrix in exhibit 5.3:

1. Companies in the upper-left quadrant exhibit strong strategic thinking and manage their operations well.
2. Companies in the upper-right quadrant have been successful through good operational management, but they cannot articulate where they are going.
3. Companies in the lower-left quadrant are excellent strategic thinkers, but they cannot implement their visions and generally are weak operationally.
4. Companies in the lower-right quadrant exhibit the worst of both dimensions and usually do not survive very long.

Robert suggests that strategic thinking skills are underdeveloped because most managers and board members have risen to the top ranks based on their skills in operations. In the course of their career development, these individuals did not naturally develop the strategic

Exhibit 5.3: The Strategic Thinking Matrix

STRATEGY (What)

		+	−
OPERATIONS (How)	**+**	EXPLICIT STRATEGIC VISION Operationally Competent	UNCERTAIN STRATEGIC VISION Operationally Competent
	−	EXPLICIT STRATEGIC VISION Operationally Incompetent	UNCERTAIN STRATEGIC VISION Operationally Incompetent

Source: Robert (1998). Reproduced with permission of The McGraw-Hill Companies.

skills necessary to help lead their companies, and minimal training or support in those areas was provided to them.

THINKING DIFFERENTLY

Gary Hamel and C. K. Prahalad (1995) state that "to have a share in the future, a company must learn to think differently about three things: 1. the meaning of competitiveness, 2. the measuring of strategy, and 3. the meaning of organization. . . . In many companies, strategic planning is essentially incremental tactical planning punctuated by heroic, and usually ill-conceived, investments. . . . To avoid this situation, we need a concept of strategy that goes beyond form filling and blank check writing."

Hamel and Prahalad argue that strategic planning, as practiced in nearly all organizations, leads to incremental change at best, small gains in market share, and pursuit of modestly profitable niches. Strategic planning is far too focused on *what is*, rather than *what could be*. Deep debates or serious consideration of radical expansion of the boundaries of existing businesses rarely occur, and strategic planning fails to stretch far enough or question fundamental assumptions of the company and its senior staff. Given the rapid rate of change in most industries, strategic planning as described in the previous section is of marginal benefit. Hamel and Prahalad (1995) call for a more exploratory and less ritualistic planning process.

In a later publication, Hamel (1998) contends that there are five ways in which more insightful strategy might be brought forth:

1. Involve new voices in the conversation about strategy, including younger employees, new employees, and others outside the inner circle of senior leadership.
2. Create new conversations about strategy, involving diverse perspectives that cut across the usual organizational boundaries.

3. Ignite new passions among individuals involved in the change process that relate to their desires to grow professionally, share in the rewards of success, and have an instrumental role in creating a unique and exciting future.
4. Develop new perspectives about the company, its businesses, its competitors, and its customers that encourage new opportunities to emerge.
5. Encourage new experiments, particularly small-scale forays into new markets and businesses, to gain insights and learning about what strategies might work and which will not.

Above all, Hamel (1998, 8) believes that senior staff must spend less time working on developing the perfect strategy and more time creating the conditions that could lead to strategy innovation: "In a discontinuous world, strategy innovation is the key to wealth creation. Strategy innovation is the capacity to reconceive the existing industry model in ways that create new value for customers, wrong-foot competitors, and produce new wealth for shareholders." The companies that have grown most successfully in the past decade or so have either invented new industries or dramatically reinvented existing ones. Their strategy is nonlinear.

In an earlier article, Hamel (1996) characterizes linear strategy as ritualistic, reductionist, extrapolative, positioning, elitist, and easy. In exceptional (and unusual) companies the strategy is inquisitive, expansive, prescient, inventive, inclusive, and demanding. Hamel suggests that strategy making must become subversive and lead to revolution, not evolution, if it is to be an effective mechanism for leading change.

Eric Beinhocker and Sarah Kaplan (2002) provide a similar attack on conventional strategic planning and a call for new ways to reinvigorate strategic planning through improved strategic thinking processes. In an article whose title, "Tired of Strategic Planning," resonates with many senior executives, they note that "many CEOs complain that their strategic-planning process yields few new ideas and is often fraught with politics" (Beinhocker and Kaplan 2002, 1). They assert that, consistent with Hamel's (1996) observations, a new process to make strategy is required. This process should have two primary goals:

1. *To build prepared minds.* If senior leaders gain a strong understanding of the business, the current and possible future environment, and the rationale for the organizational direction agreed on through the strategic planning process, they are more likely to be able to respond swiftly and effectively to challenges and opportunities that emerge.

2. *To build creative minds.* Beinhocker and Kaplan (2002) agree with Hamel (1996) that strategic experimentation is appropriate and allows for controlled testing of potential future opportunities. They also agree that many of the issues that companies face today are best addressed in multidisciplinary, crosscutting forums that demand new voices, discussions, and perspectives.

Two recent articles provide concrete, practical advice on how to insert strategic thinking into the management routines of an organization. Freek Vermeulen (2015) says there are five big questions organizational leaders need to ask regularly:

1. *What does not fit?* Are there business units that are peripheral and don't add (or even may detract from) significant value to the organization?

2. *What would an outsider do?* If new external people were in charge, would they jettison legacy products, projects, or beliefs?

3. *Is my organization consistent with my strategy?* Is the company structured to execute the strategy effectively?
4. *Do I understand why we do it this way?* Are practices, habits, operations, processes, and systems appropriate for successful strategy execution?
5. *What might be the long-term consequences?* Have we evaluated the possible substantive effects of this strategy in the long run?

Michael Birshan and Jayanti Kar (2012) suggest a few other basic devices to become more strategic. With the pace of change accelerating in all industries, being on the lookout for potential disrupters must become a regular part of strategic leadership. Technology and new competitors are the most frequent and obvious sources of disruption. Part of good strategic thinking is developing an early warning system to identify emerging disruptors. In terms of translating strategic insights into effective action, time spent devising innovative ways to communicate strategy—ways that will break through the postmillennial information glut—is critical.

NEW APPROACHES TO PROMOTING STRATEGIC THINKING

Businesses outside healthcare are years ahead of the healthcare sector in promoting strategic thinking in their organizations. Many companies use the following approaches:

- Contingency planning to address a single uncertainty in a given situation
- Sensitivity analysis to examine the effect of a change in one variable while all other variables remain constant
- Simulation to analyze the effects of simultaneous change in multiple variables

Scenario Planning

Healthcare increasingly employs an even more robust approach: scenario planning. In contrast to contingency planning and sensitivity analysis, scenario planning allows for multiple changes in variables, incorporating both objective analysis (which characterizes simulation) and subjective considerations (which are commonly found in two narrower approaches, contingency planning and sensitivity analysis).

According to Paul J. H. Schoemaker (1995, 27), "Scenario planning attempts to capture the richness and range of possibilities, stimulating decision makers to consider changes they would otherwise ignore. At the same time, it organizes those possibilities into narratives that are easier to grasp and use than great volumes of data."

Schoemaker indicates that scenario planning is particularly beneficial for organizations facing the following conditions:

- Uncertainty is high relative to managers' ability to predict or adjust.
- Many costly surprises have occurred in the past.
- The company does not perceive or generate new opportunities.
- The quality of strategic thinking is low (i.e., too routine, too bureaucratic).
- The industry has experienced significant change or is about to.
- The company wants a common language and framework that doesn't stifle diversity.
- There are strong differences of opinion, with multiple opinions having merit.
- The company's competitors are using scenario planning.

Schoemaker observes that because scenarios are designed to construct possible futures but not specific strategies for dealing with them, some organizations find it beneficial to involve outsiders, such as major customers, key suppliers, regulators, consultants, and academics, in the scenario development process. The objective is "to build a shared framework for strategic thinking that encourages diversity and sharper perceptions about external changes and opportunities" (Schoemaker 1995, 28).

Schoemaker suggests a ten-step approach to scenario development:

1. Define the scope of scenarios to be developed, including time horizon and range. Look at past sources of uncertainty and volatility as guides.
2. Identify the major stakeholders who could influence the range of considerations defined in step 1.
3. Describe key future trends likely to affect the issues identified in step 1.
4. Identify major uncertainties that could significantly affect each issue.
5. Construct initial scenario themes.
6. Check for consistency and plausibility and revise scenario outlines as necessary.
7. Develop learning scenarios or the first full-scale version of the scenarios.
8. Identify research needs to flesh out uncertainties, trends, and blind spots in the learning scenarios.
9. Develop quantitative models, as appropriate, to better examine the interactions of certain variables.
10. Evolve toward discussion scenarios, through an iterative process, to converge on the final scenarios that will be used to test strategies to develop new ideas.

Moreover, Schoemaker believes that good scenarios meet four tests: they are relevant, internally consistent, long term in perspective, and describe clearly different futures.

Decision Analysis and Game Theory

Marion C. Jennings, Scott B. Clay, and Erin P. Carr (2000) advocate decision analysis and game theory as two additional techniques that have been used in business for many years to address future uncertainties creatively. While scenario planning is an excellent approach to addressing a large number of uncertainties, decision analysis works well when a limited number of possible alternatives exist. Game theory allows understanding of interdependencies among affected parties as a result of strategic initiatives, especially the reactions of competitors, strategic alliance partners, customers, and suppliers. These approaches are appropriate in many situations routinely encountered in strategic analysis and should become basic tools in the near future.

Blue Ocean Strategy

W. Chan Kim and Renée Mauborgne's (2005) research led to the coining of the term *blue ocean strategy* to describe the creation of uncontested market space. They argue that most companies pursue incremental improvements by attempting to outcompete their competitors and, in a zero-sum game, increase their share of a crowded market. The more successful approach is to expand the boundaries of their market or invent entirely new market space (the blue ocean).

These innovators do not use the competition as a reference point, but instead follow a different strategic logic they term *value innovation*. Value innovation, which defies the conventional competitive paradigm of having to choose between differentiation and cost, combines these two options to find new and uncontested market space (see exhibits 5.4 and 5.5). Value innovation is created in the market space where a company's actions favorably affect both its cost structure and its value proposition to buyers. Cost savings are made by eliminating and reducing the factors on which an industry

Exhibit 5.4: Value Innovation: The Cornerstone of Blue Ocean Strategy

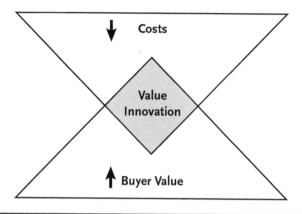

Source: Kim and Mauborgne (2005).

competes. Buyer value is lifted by raising and creating elements the industry has never offered. Over time, costs are reduced further as scale economies kick in because of the high sales volumes that superior value generates.

This new space creates opportunities for rapid and profitable growth, unlike the *red ocean* in which nearly all companies operate and compete. Kim and Mauborgne cite many examples of companies applying this kind of strategic thinking to the problem of crowded markets—Cirque du Soleil in the circus business is one example.

Kim and Mauborgne advise that blue ocean strategy contrasts with traditional strategic planning in the following ways:

- It draws on collective wisdom, unlike top-down or bottom-up planning.
- It focuses on building the big picture more than on number crunching.
- It should be conversational rather than documentation driven.
- It must be creative, rather than largely analytical.

Exhibit 5.5: Red Ocean Versus Blue Ocean Strategy

Red Ocean Strategy	Blue Ocean Strategy
Compete in existing market space.	Create uncontested market space.
Beat the competition.	Make the competition irrelevant.
Exploit existing demand.	Create and capture new demand.
Make the value–cost trade-off.	Break the value–cost trade-off.
Align the whole system of a firm's activities with its strategic choice of differentiation or low cost.	Align the whole system of a firm's activities in pursuit of differentiation and low cost.

Source: Kim and Mauborgne (2005).

- It should be motivational (resulting in "willing commitment"), instead of bargaining driven (resulting in "negotiated commitment").

The bottom line, in their view, is to focus on how to break away from the competition and create blue ocean space, then layer in the details of how to implement the strategy.

Advanced Strategic Thinking

Academic and business journals present a growing body of literature on what could be characterized as *advanced strategic thinking* for professionals who have a desire to learn more. The work of Hanford (1995) is representative of this body of work. Hanford developed a program called Tools for Thinking Strategically (TTS), which is a skills-building and training program on this topic for trustees and executives. Hanford's program is designed to perform several functions:

- Redefine or confirm the director's and executive's high-level role of setting direction by looking "outward, upward, and forward" to implement major changes and improvements

- Establish skills to formulate and successfully implement effective policies and strategies
- Develop a comfort level with assuming radically different behaviors
- Develop agility and adeptness in moving between strategic and operational behaviors by knowing when to be "in your helicopter" (acting strategically) versus being "on the ground" (acting operationally)
- Assist individuals in becoming more personally effective in a variety of strategic-support skill areas
- Build confidence about the ability to think strategically
- Achieve constancy in strategic thinking as a result of more competence and confidence

Hanford also identifies four basic strategic thinking tools available to trustees and executives to enable them to think better in order to direct and manage better (exhibit 5.6):

1. *Thinking skills*, in which Hanford identifies four subtools:
   - Reframing, or developing one or more optional approaches to addressing an issue or opportunity (often by shifting the focus) rather than falling victim to "there's only one way to go."
   - Mapmaking, a deliberate approach to developing a full range of alternatives for addressing an issue before deciding what to do about it; this activity is accompanied by a collaborative approach—which includes developing the map and then deciding what to do about it—rather than the typical adversarial senior group discussion and decision-making process.
   - Using searching questions to stimulate discussions of the "what ifs" and "why nots" in confronting the big issues facing the organization.

Exhibit 5.6: Tools for Thinking Strategically

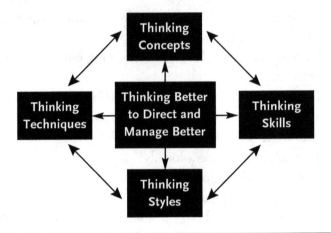

Source: Hanford (1995) in Garratt (1995). Reproduced with permission of The McGraw-Hill Companies.

- Asking effective questions when reviewing issues in order to enhance creativity, increase commitment to organizational goals, and empower others to maximize their contributions to organizational success and their own job satisfaction.

2. *Thinking concepts*, in which Hanford identifies three subtools:
   - Holistic thinking to expand the breadth of individual and group thinking, based on the premise that the more fully you think about a situation, the better you can manage it
   - Deeper thinking through the realization that results are dependent not only on effective actions but also on values, beliefs, and assumptions
   - An expanded range of content thinking. Most director and executive content thinking can be categorized as "either/or" thinking (it is either *x* or *y*); expand the

range of alternatives to include "more/less" and "both/ and" thinking. Similarly, most director and executive process thinking is "stay put" thinking, which is fine for straightforward issues in stable situations; expand the range of alternatives to include "minor from/to" and "major from/to" thinking.

3. *Thinking techniques*, in which Hanford identifies four subtools:
   - "Both/and," which involves thinking about or explicit recognition of potential inconsistencies or trade-offs in decision making and then the creation of a map of a dilemma—a tool that can generate some approaches to resolution.
   - Mind mapping, a process that identifies the essential elements of a strategic challenge and the interrelationships among the elements, which facilitates planning to meet the challenge.
   - Effective prioritization to reduce the number of important issues, based on urgency, relevance, growth, and ease of implementation, and to focus organizational resources on these priorities.
   - Choices and consequences thinking (also known as "more/less" thinking), a technique that involves purposefully identifying alternative courses of action and then determining the relative merit of each alternative.

4. *Thinking styles*, in which Hanford identifies three subtools:
   - Revealing thinking intentions (or how you go about thinking). There are three basic thinking intentions: realize a new idea, describe what is true, or judge what is right. Recognizing this form of tunnel thinking allows development of an enriched and more balanced style for better decision making.
   - Identifying a leader's member type. There are five types—synthesist, idealist, pragmatist, analyst, or

realist. This tool expands thinking behavior to enhance decision making.
- Understanding learning styles to improve how leaders learn, and promoting continuous improvement based on continuous learning.

Those who wish to know more about these concepts would benefit greatly from reading the source material on which this synopsis is based and then experimenting with one or more of the subtools. Ellen F. Goldman (2007) has also written extensively about how strategic thinking capabilities develop and how executives might become better strategic thinkers; her work is a cornerstone reference in this area.

CONCLUSION

Material presented in this chapter presents new approaches and behaviors, as well as some long-standing techniques, to enhance strategic planning in healthcare organizations. It should be considered for adoption, especially given the increasing rate and pace of change in the field. In conclusion, this comment from the CEO of a large, global bank captures the essence of the shift in perspective expressed in this chapter: "It is very easy for someone in my position to be very busy all the time. There is always another meeting you really have to attend, and you can fly somewhere else pretty much every other day. However, I feel that that is not what I am paid to do. It is my job to carefully think about our strategy" (Vermeulen 2015, 1).

REFERENCES

Beinhocker, E. D., and S. Kaplan. 2002. "Tired of Strategic Planning?" *McKinsey Quarterly*, June, 1–7.

Birshan, M., and J. Kar. 2012. "Becoming More Strategic: Three Tips for Any Executive." *McKinsey Quarterly*, July, 1–7.

Garratt, R. (ed.). 1995. *Developing Strategic Thought: Rediscovering the Art of Direction-Giving*. London: McGraw-Hill.

Ginter, P. M., W. J. Duncan, and L. E. Swayne. 2013. *Strategic Management of Health Care Organizations*, 7th ed. San Francisco: Jossey-Bass.

Goldman, E. F. 2007. "Strategic Thinking at the Top." *MIT Sloan Management Review* 48 (4): 75–81.

Hamel, G. 1998. "Strategy Innovation and the Quest for Value." *Sloan Management Review* 39 (2): 7–14.

———. 1996. "Strategy as Revolution." *Harvard Business Review*, July–August, 69–82.

Hamel, G., and C. K. Prahalad. 1995. "Thinking Differently." *Business Quarterly* 59 (4): 22–35.

Hanford, P. 1995. "Developing Director and Executive Competencies in Strategic Thinking." In *Developing Strategic Thought: Rediscovering the Art of Direction-Giving*, edited by B. Garratt, 157–84. London: McGraw-Hill.

———. 1983. "Managing for Results." Unpublished paper written for the Public Service Board, Queensland State Government, Brisbane, Australia.

Hickman, C., and M. Silva. 1984. "On Becoming a Strategic Thinker." In *Creating Excellence: Managing Corporate Culture, Strategy, and Change in the New Age*. London: Allen & Unwin.

Jennings, M., S. B. Clay, and E. P. Carr. 2000. "Tools to Address Uncertainty." In *Health Care Strategy for Uncertain Times*, edited by M. Jennings, 99–134. San Francisco: Jossey-Bass.

Kaufman, R. 1991. *Strategic Planning Plus: An Organization Guide.* Newbury Park, CA: SAGE Publications.

Kim, W. C., and R. Mauborgne. 2005. *Blue Ocean Strategy: How to Create Uncontested Market Space and Make Competition Irrelevant.* Boston: Harvard Business Review Press.

Mintzberg, H. 1994. "The Fall and Rise of Strategic Planning." *Harvard Business Review*, January–February, 107–13.

Porter, M. E. 1987. "The State of Strategic Thinking." *The Economist*, May 23, 18.

Robert, M. 1998. *Strategy Pure and Simple II: How Winning Companies Dominate Their Competitors*, rev. ed. New York: McGraw-Hill.

Rumelt, R. 2011. *Good Strategy, Bad Strategy: The Difference and Why It Matters*. New York: Crown Business.

Schoemaker, P. J. H. 1995. "Scenario Planning: A Tool for Strategic Thinking." *Sloan Management Review* 36 (2): 25–41.

Vermeulen, F. 2015. "5 Strategy Questions Every Leader Should Make Time For." *Harvard Business Review*. Published September 3. https://hbr.org/2015/09/5-strategy-questions-every-leader-should-make-time-for.

The Strategic Planning Process

CHAPTER 6

Phase 1: Analyzing the Environment

In God we trust. All others bring data.

—*Edward Deming*

You can never plan the future by the past.

—*Edmund Burke*

LOOKING FORWARD VERSUS LOOKING BACKWARD

Strategic planning typically begins with an analysis of the current situation and recent history of the organization, referred to as the *situation analysis* or *environmental assessment* (see exhibit 6.1).

The environmental assessment should

- identify past successes and failures: what has worked, what has not, and why;
- give trustees and others less knowledgeable about the organization a solid grounding for constructive involvement;
- help determine what factors are subject to the organization's control and influence; and
- identify how external forces might affect the organization in the future.

Exhibit 6.1: Developing the Plan: Environmental Assessment

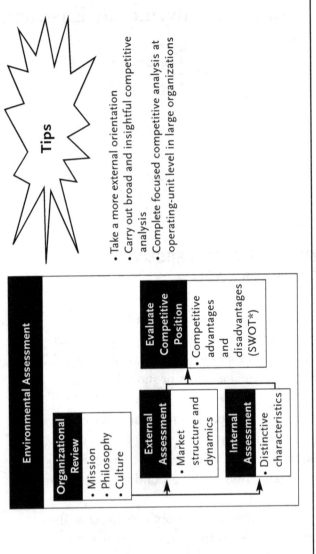

Tips

- Take a more external orientation
- Carry out broad and insightful competitive analysis
- Complete focused competitive analysis at operating-unit level in large organizations

Environmental Assessment

Organizational Review
- Mission
- Philosophy
- Culture

External Assessment
- Market structure and dynamics

Internal Assessment
- Distinctive characteristics

Evaluate Competitive Position
- Competitive advantages and disadvantages (SWOT*)

*SWOT = strengths, weaknesses, opportunities, and threats.
© 2017 Veralon Partners Inc.

Although the environmental assessment may be viewed as mere busywork for the planning staff before real strategic planning begins, it has valid and important purposes that should be enumerated and highlighted at the start of the assessment. Among them, as the first activity in the planning process, the environmental assessment largely sets the tone for the strategic plan and indicates how the rest of the planning process is likely to unfold by examining the following questions:

- Will the process be comprehensive in scope?
- Which key organizational stakeholders will be involved in a constructive way?
- Will it be highly structured or loosely organized?
- Will it be driven by facts, strive to overcome bias, and focus on critical issues?
- Have the outputs of the strategic planning process been clearly articulated, and will this process drive toward their achievement?
- Is a planning schedule being followed, and will that planning lead to action?

As discussed in chapter 3, many planning efforts get off to a poor start because the planning process and activities lack sufficient advance conceptualization, organization, or explanation to the whole organization. The environmental assessment, if poorly planned and executed, can derail subsequent strategic planning activities. The environmental assessment is characterized by three separate processes: information gathering, distillation of key findings, and translation into conclusions.

Perhaps the most common concern when undertaking an environmental assessment is that the staff may become enmeshed in data gathering and analysis, bogging down the entire planning process early—a problem known as analysis paralysis. Guidelines and resources for effectively carrying out data gathering—a complicated and controversial task—are provided in exhibits 6.2, 6.3, and 6.4.

Exhibit 6.2: Minimum Data Requirements for the Environmental Assessment

Internal	External
• Characteristics and utilization of major programs and services • Key indicators: facilities, equipment, and staff • Financial performance and position	• Major demographic and economic indicators • Major technology, reimbursement, and regulatory factors • Position of major programs and services • Profile and analysis of key competitors • Future market size and characteristics

© 2017 Veralon Partners Inc.

While it is important to compile a database that clearly reflects the organization's historical performance and market, strategic planning is not primarily an exercise in plotting historical patterns and then extrapolating. As the Burke quote at the beginning of this chapter implies, historical performance is not a reliable indicator of the future. Reviewing recent history and analyzing successes and failures is a comforting activity. But organizations gain little from overanalysis of the past, and whatever momentum and excitement it may be able to create at the initiation of strategic planning will likely be lost if historical performance, particularly negative trends or areas of underperformance, becomes the major focus of the strategic planning process.

Being deliberate and focused in both the type and volume of data that are being sought will not only expedite the environmental assessment but also ensure excessive time and resources are not spent overanalyzing information simply because it is available. A few tips for organizing the data collection process follow:

Exhibit 6.3: Online Healthcare Data Resources

- Agency for Healthcare Research and Quality — www.ahrq.gov
- American Hospital Association — www.aha.org
- American Medical Association — www.ama-assn.org
- Center for Consumer Information and Insurance Oversight — www.cms.gov/CCIIO
- Centers for Disease Control and Prevention — www.cdc.gov
- Centers for Medicare & Medicaid Services — www.medicare.gov/hospitalcompare www.medicare.gov/nursinghomecompare
- The Dartmouth Atlas of Health Care — www.dartmouthatlas.org
- Health Resources and Services Administration — www.hrsa.gov
- Kaiser Family Foundation — www.kff.org
- National Cancer Institute — www.cancer.gov
- National Center for Health Statistics — www.cdc.gov/nchs
- State-specific hospital discharge databases — (Varies by state)

Exhibit 6.4: Creative Data Gathering for the Environmental Assessment: Competitor Intelligence

Hard Data	Soft Data
• State licensure and other state filings • 990 and 10-K reports and other federal filings • Hospital associations • Public vendors	• Annual reports • Websites • Public relations releases or brochures • Press releases • Presentations by executives • Former employees

© 2017 Veralon Partners Inc.

- Create a checklist prior to data collection identifying the specific categories of information that will be most helpful for the organization and situation.
- Limit the historical data to three to five years of trend information.
- Use existing or regularly updated data sets, particularly those that are commonly employed in the organization, as they are more likely to be accurate and are easier to obtain than customized reports.
- Select appropriate benchmarks for comparison.
- Inventory information as it is collected and be sure to clearly label files (e.g., type of information, years included) so information can be easily located and accessed later in the strategic planning process.

While quantitative analytics can tell much about *how* an organization has performed in recent years, data in isolation lack context and perspective on *why* the organization chose a particular path or what environmental factors affected performance. Stakeholder interviews provide valuable insights that will support or supplement data findings. These interviews also shed light on topics that cannot be extracted from analytics, such as culture or an organization's readiness for change (exhibit 6.5). Board members, senior management, and physician leaders are typically the subjects of these interviews. Interviews should not be limited to internal stakeholders. External constituents, including regional competitors' senior management, major payer representatives, community leaders, and relevant political representatives, can offer perspectives as to how the organization is perceived in the market.

If more extensive feedback is desired or required, online surveys or focus groups can be useful tools to engage a broader group of stakeholders. Although the substantive value of input gathering may diminish significantly as greater amounts of information are collected, the political value of soliciting and carefully listening to organizational leaders' and stakeholders' opinions should not be ignored.

Exhibit 6.5: Internal and External Interview Topics

Internal Interview Topics	External Interview Topics
• Perceived strengths and weaknesses • Recent or planned initiatives • Strategic priorities • Desired future state or vision	• Community perception or reputation of the organization • Local or regional market trends • Needed services in the community

© 2017 Veralon Partners Inc.

APPROACH TO THE ORGANIZATIONAL ASSESSMENT

The organizational assessment combines data analysis with qualitative information to formulate an accurate profile of the historical performance of the organization. Along with the market assessment, discussed in the next section, it establishes the organization's strengths, weaknesses, opportunities, and threats (SWOT) and identifies competitive advantages and disadvantages that serve as a springboard for subsequent strategic planning activities.

Telling the story of a complex organization is challenging. Information needs to be organized in a way that allows conclusions to be extracted and easily understood by various constituencies. It is helpful to group information into summary categories. These categories and the data that are evaluated will be different for every organization. Exhibit 6.6 shows possible categories that can be explored, and related key questions that should be answered in the organizational assessment.

Larger, complex organizations may need to evaluate entities or lines of business separately, while smaller organizations may be able to consider the enterprise as a whole. For example, a large health system might profile its acute care business, medical group,

Exhibit 6.6: Possible Information Summary Categories

Scale and scope of services	• What is the organization's coverage of the care continuum? • What is the organization's size (revenue and volume) relative to competitors? • What are the breadth and depth of services? • What are the number, nature, and distribution of customer access points? • How is utilization trending by service or entity?
Financials	• What is the current financial position? • What has been the recent financial performance and what are the drivers of that performance? • What is the organization's payer mix? • What types of reimbursement contracts are currently in place and what are being proposed? • Have any major capital needs been identified?
Providers	• What is the profile of the medical staff and other providers (e.g., number, age mix)? • What is the base of employed or tightly aligned providers? • What is the degree of provider engagement?
Value	• How does the organization perform on clinical quality, patient safety, and patient satisfaction measures? • What is the cost of care or service delivery? • How are services priced?
Integration	• Do elements of the organization effectively coordinate care or service delivery? • Are organizational goals and incentives aligned across departments or entities? • Is there significant "leakage" or internal referrals to external entities?
Operations	• How efficient is the organization? • Are there any significant facility or staffing needs? • How is the organization positioned in information technology?

(continued)

(continued from previous page)

Competitive position or market capture	• What is the organization's market share by service and geography? • Who is the market leader by service and geography? • Is there significant outmigration from the service area for any service or consumer group?
Future orientation	• What is the organization's reliance on inpatient and fee-for-service revenue? • Can the organization manage change? • What is the organization's structure, and does that structure support future growth?

© 2017 Veralon Partners Inc.

post-acute care business, health plan, and so on individually across relevant categories.

The Organizational Assessment's End Product

The product of the organizational assessment should be a summary of the results that contains a limited number of charts and tables that are both clear and concise in their key conclusions. (See exhibits 6.7 and 6.8 for examples.) These conclusions should not simply describe trend information but rather explore implications for the organization's position moving forward. These implications can range from an urgent or immediate need for attention to a source of competitive advantage in any given category. Supporting documentation is required and should be prepared and available as backup. No exact measure for how much supporting documentation is necessary exists, as every organizational assessment is unique. A guiding rule is that if a potential table, graph, or analysis does not support or answer a key question identified in the organizational assessment, it is likely extraneous.

Exhibit 6.7: Snapshot of an Integrated System's Health Plan, 2017

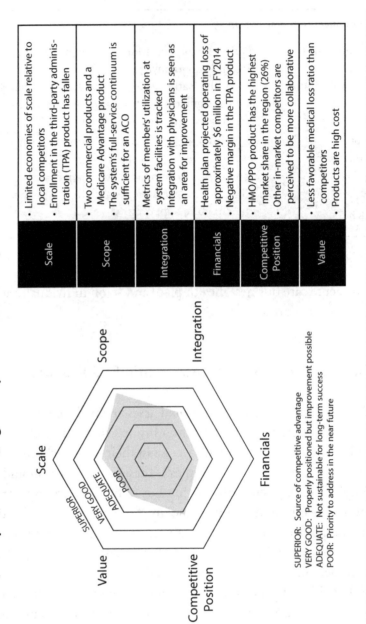

Scale	• Limited economies of scale relative to local competitors • Enrollment in the third-party administration (TPA) product has fallen
Scope	• Two commercial products and a Medicare Advantage product • The system's full-service continuum is sufficient for an ACO
Integration	• Metrics of members' utilization at system facilities is tracked • Integration with physicians is seen as an area for improvement
Financials	• Health plan projected operating loss of approximately $6 million in FY2014 • Negative margin in the TPA product
Competitive Position	• HMO/PPO product has the highest market share in the region (26%) • Other in-market competitors are perceived to be more collaborative
Value	• Less favorable medical loss ratio than competitors • Products are high cost

SUPERIOR: Source of competitive advantage
VERY GOOD: Properly positioned but improvement possible
ADEQUATE: Not sustainable for long-term success
POOR: Priority to address in the near future

© 2017 Veralon Partners Inc.

Exhibit 6.8: Community Hospital's Organizational Assessment, 2017

Categories	Assessment Focus	Urgent Need for Medical Attention	Major Changes Required for Long-term Stability	On the Right Track; Needs Additional Development for Continued Success	Well-positioned for Long-term Success with Minor Gaps	Well-positioned for Current and Future Competitive Advantage
Scale/scope	– Relative size of operations – Mix and distribution of services and site – Care continuum coverage				★	
Financial position	– Current and historical financial performance, position, and access to capital		★			
Market position	– Current and historic market share performance and position			★		
Value position	– Quality and service outcomes relative to cost and price		★			
Integration	– Physician alignment – Coordination among services and sites within the system – Care continuum integration	★				

© 2017 Veralon Partners Inc.

APPROACH TO THE MARKET ASSESSMENT

The market assessment, like the organizational assessment, should be an accurate profile of the organization's historical performance as it relates to the marketplace. The external assessment profiles the historical performance and evolution of the marketplace and initiates the process of looking forward by explicitly considering market trends and forecasts. The external assessment has four main components.

Review Population Characteristics

This task identifies the broadest trends and variables that have had and will have an impact on organizational performance. While key community demographic, economic, and health status indicators for the past three to five years should be profiled and forecasts provided for the next five to ten years, if available, it is important to note that minor shifts in these measures are of minimal or no consequence to the strategic planning process. Organizations should take care not to overreach and instead should aim to complete a review with a scope that is general and high level rather than detailed. In addition to identifying broad trends, this analysis is occasionally useful in identifying geographical areas or population segments with strong potential for future cultivation.

Review the State of Healthcare Delivery in the Local and Regional Market

This step is perhaps the most important in the market assessment and should be afforded requisite attention and resources. The purpose of reviewing applicable healthcare technology, delivery, reimbursement, regulatory, consolidation, teaching, and research trends is to identify any major environmental influences that have affected recent organizational performance and, more important, may affect future performance and strategies. (Examples of such reviews for two areas in the United States are shown in exhibits 6.9 and 6.10.)

In addition to identifying an anticipated trend's impact on organizational performance, key statistics or research should be included as support for the conclusions.

Exhibit 6.9: Select Market Characteristics in Central North Carolina, 2015

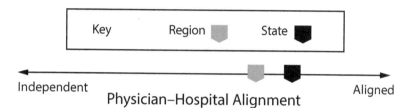

Independent — Physician–Hospital Alignment — Aligned

Majority of physicians in the region employed by integrated delivery systems or affiliated with ACOs or large, independent, multispecialty groups; several independent primary care groups
NC has a higher physician employment rate than the US average (by 16 percentage points)

Fragmented — Hospital Consolidation — Consolidated

Regional/state market characterized by medium to large regional and multistate systems
82% of hospitals in the state affiliated/owned by a system, as compared to 62% in the US

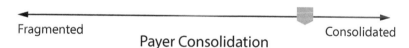

Fragmented — Payer Consolidation — Consolidated

Individual, small group, and large group markets dominated Insurer A
Much higher than average proportion of covered lives in individual market (vs. large or small group)

© 2017 Veralon Partners Inc.

Analyze Competitors

Analyzing competitors is another critical task—and often the most difficult one. Competitor data in healthcare can be incomplete and out-of-date, although good information can be collected with some hard work and resourcefulness.

Exhibit 6.10: Select Market Characteristics in Southern Indiana, 2015

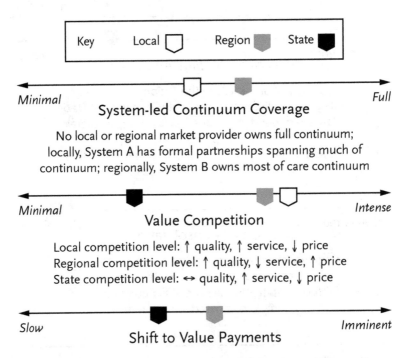

Key   Local ☐   Region ■   State ■

System-led Continuum Coverage
Minimal ←————————————————→ Full

No local or regional market provider owns full continuum; locally, System A has formal partnerships spanning much of continuum; regionally, System B owns most of care continuum

Value Competition
Minimal ←————————————————→ Intense

Local competition level: ↑ quality, ↑ service, ↓ price
Regional competition level: ↑ quality, ↓ service, ↑ price
State competition level: ↔ quality, ↑ service, ↓ price

Shift to Value Payments
Slow ←————————————————→ Imminent

State: Low IN HMO penetration rate vs. US (17% vs. 24%); mediocre IN and KY performance on Medicare value-based payments, 30-day readmissions

Region: High relative fee-for-service prices signal likely future rate cuts; Insurer A implementation of wrap payments in IN will solidify footholds and accelerate shift; moderate accountable care organization penetration

© 2017 Veralon Partners Inc.

Competitors may operate on a variety of levels. Some organizations may compete in most or all service categories, whereas others may do so in one or a few select niches. An increasingly common mistake in competitor assessments, particularly for hospitals and health systems, is an exclusive focus on traditional competitors. In many markets across the United States, new market entrants are competing with acute care providers, particularly in the retail space.

Collect competitor data from local, regional, state, and national sources, including those listed in exhibits 6.3 and 6.4. Because of this topic's importance, and because of evidence that many healthcare organizations have historically failed to complete this task adequately, a three-part example from a strategic plan (exhibits 6.11, 6.12, 6.13) demonstrates a rigorous analysis for a fictional organization.

Market Forecasts and Implications

In addition to assessing anticipated population, economic, and health status changes in the market, it may be necessary to forecast health services utilization. This step is not always required and can constitute over-analysis in some circumstances. Utilization forecasts can be employed if there is a predetermined consensus that the strategic plan will likely focus on a specific segment of services (e.g., outpatient services, cancer services) and will necessitate more thorough analysis. The forecast will include a baseline level of market utilization for the specific services and projected growth or reduction of those services based on a variety of factors, including population and demographic changes, variations in care delivery (e.g., surgeries shifting to outpatient settings), or the effect of efforts to manage care to reduce avoidable admissions.

The External Assessment's End Product

A summary of the market structure and dynamics should be prepared in parallel form to that of the internal assessment. When possible, comparison to benchmarks can help focus the summary

Exhibit 6.11: Analysis of XYZ's Competitors' Strategies, 2017

Strategy	System A	System B	AMC A	AMC B	Comm. Hospital	Niche Provider
Value position	✪	O	O	O	●	●
Market capture	✪	●	●	✪	O	✪
Horizontal integration (w/ other health systems)	✪	●	●	✪	●	O
Vertical integration (w/ payers and physicians)	✪	O	O	✪	O	O
GME and research	O	O	✪	✪	O	O
Marketing and consumer preferences	✪	O	●	✪	O	●

Symbol	Description
✪	High risk to XYZ
●	Moderate risk to XYZ
O	Low risk to XYZ

System A and AMC B are XYZ's most significant competitors

© 2017 Veralon Partners Inc.

on noteworthy key points. A brief report with several charts and tables accompanied by modest narration or highlighting of key points should suffice. Additional materials may be available for backup support if needed.

TRANSLATION INTO CONCLUSIONS

The internal and external assessments need to produce three main outputs to lay the foundation for subsequent activities: (1) a succinct, pointed, and honest statement of the organization's competitive advantages and disadvantages in the marketplace; (2) assumptions about the future environment; and (3), with the content of the first

Exhibit 6.12: XYZ's Future Competitive Environment and Planning Implications, 2020

Strategy	System A	System B	AMC A	AMC B	Community Hospital	Niche Provider	Planning Implications for XYZ
Quality or cost differentiation	X				X	X	Enhance value position in core services
Targeted growth in priority geography	X		X	X		X	Strengthen existing referral relationships in priority geography
Network development	X			X			Build and integrate care continuum
Survival mode		X					Consider candidates for affiliation or acquisition

XYZ will face difficult competition in its target geography and will need to be active in network development to keep pace with the scale development of its most significant

Exhibit 6.13: Potential Future Competitor Positioning Re: XYZ, 2017–2020

Organization	Baseline Forecast	Aggressive Forecast (in Addition to Baseline)	Declining Forecast
System A	• Continues ambulatory growth • Employs significant number of independent physicians • Adds 1–2 community hospitals to system	• Establishes insurance product • Develops significant base of covered lives • National prominence for clinical integration or other innovations	• Federal Trade Commission challenges merger • Becomes overextended and pulls back on investments and programs
System B	• Remains strong in its core services • Modest growth attributed to physician practice acquisition	• Out-of-market parent system infuses major capital resources • Develops integrated service lines	• Financial erosion to a safety-net hospital
Community hospital	• Affiliates with local system • Capital infusion boosts select services	• Affiliates with AMC B to establish strong academic–community network	• Does not draw affiliation interest and reduces scope of services or closes
Etc.	Etc.	Etc.	Etc.

two outputs in mind, identification of critical planning issues that require resolution in the strategic planning process.

Competitive Advantages and Disadvantages

No particular approach or format for determining and displaying competitive advantages and disadvantages is universally accepted. In general, the three most reliable measures of competitive advantage or disadvantage are value position (quality relative to cost), market share, and bond rating. Upward historical trends in these variables usually indicate a strong competitive position. However, trends seen in healthcare organizations are rarely clear-cut. Simply focusing on these indicators, for example, masks major shifts in competitive position because of the lagged effect of capital or human investments.

The most commonly used format for displaying competitive advantage and disadvantage is a SWOT analysis. Each category in the analysis has a specific orientation (internal, external) and purpose for examination as shown in exhibit 6.14. A sample SWOT analysis is provided in exhibit 6.15.

While the team may initially generate a lengthy SWOT analysis, the final list should be refined to a one-page summary. As the exhibits show, items may be drawn from any category of the internal and external assessments, but not every assessment category needs to be represented in the final summary.

The purpose of the SWOT analysis is to provide organizational leadership with a clear assessment of where the organizational stands in its competitive marketplace. Little benefit is derived from applying overly complicated analysis to achieve the results. Leadership must use its skills, experience, and judgment to synthesize all of the external assessment findings and determine the organization's real advantages and disadvantages.

Assumptions About the Future

Up to this point in its process, the environmental assessment has been concerned primarily with the past. The remainder of the assessment and the strategic planning process shifts the focus to the future.

The first forward-looking task is to develop a picture of the future environment, at least three to five years hence and perhaps further, in which the organization will operate. This forecast should consider key external factors (some local or regional, others state or national)

Exhibit 6.14: SWOT Category Orientation

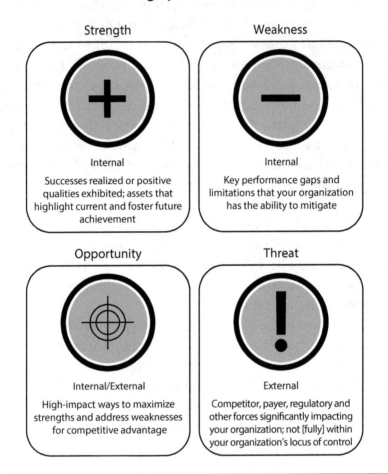

Strength

Internal

Successes realized or positive qualities exhibited; assets that highlight current and foster future achievement

Weakness

Internal

Key performance gaps and limitations that your organization has the ability to mitigate

Opportunity

Internal/External

High-impact ways to maximize strengths and address weaknesses for competitive advantage

Threat

External

Competitor, payer, regulatory and other forces significantly impacting your organization; not [fully] within your organization's locus of control

that may have a significant impact on the organization's future strategies. It should not be strictly numerical (for example, delineating market size and the precise level of reimbursement changes) but rather a qualitative and macrolevel view of significant future and external influences.

The predictions of healthcare futurists and forecasts from publications and associations that track emerging trends can help healthcare organizations formulate their own assumptions (see the suggested readings at the end of this chapter for examples of available resources). Gary Hamel and C. K. Prahalad (1994, 123) write that few organizations spend an adequate amount of time thinking about the future, noting that "senior managers devote less than 3% . . . of their time to building a *corporate* perspective on the future. In some companies, the figure is less than 1%. Our experience suggests

Exhibit 6.15: An Integrated Health System's Strategic Profile, 2015

Strengths	Weaknesses
• Facilities (hospital campuses) • Scope of services • Variety of specialized services • Medical equipment and technology • Owned health plan • Primary care base • Quality outcomes relative to competitors	• Limited debt capacity • Siloed system components • Relationship with medical staff • Condition of post-acute and ambulatory facilities • Leadership in transition • Patient satisfaction
Opportunities	**Threats**
• Rural outreach • System integration • Competitor ownership transition • Shift to customer-focused culture • University affiliation • Insurance product advancement • Affiliations • Transition to value-based environment	• Local/regional economy • Declining or flat reimbursement • Specialist alignment to other systems • Competitor market share gains • Historical perspective of the organization as non-collaborative

© 2017 Veralon Partners Inc.

that to develop a distinctive point of view about the future, senior managers must be willing to devote considerably more of their time" (emphasis in original).

Historically, healthcare organizations and the general business community have predicated much of their planning on one view of the future environment—usually a linear extrapolation from the past—rather than evaluating a wide range of possible futures. The upheavals in healthcare and other fields illustrate how this singular view of the future has led to major errors in organizational strategy and legitimate concern about the wisdom of planning for the future with a narrow view of possible future realities.

In the 1970s, General Motors failed to explore fully the impact of environmentalism, the importance of quality and speed in manufacturing, and the power of OPEC—the Organization of the Petroleum Exporting Countries (Schoemaker 1995). In the 1980s, IBM and Digital Equipment Corporation failed to account for the consequences of personal computers (Schoemaker 1995). In a more recent example, few healthcare leaders predicted the election of Donald Trump and the resulting implications for healthcare policy.

According to Hamel and Prahalad (1994, 126), "If senior executives don't have reasonably detailed answers to the 'future' questions, and if the answers they have are not significantly different from the 'today' answers, there is little chance that their companies will remain market leaders."

Planning for the future in a narrow, limited environmental context may have been acceptable in the more static, highly regulated healthcare environment that prevailed through the early 1990s. However, this approach is no longer feasible and constitutes one of the main differences between contemporary strategic planning methods and those of even the recent past.

To ensure that a broader perspective is adopted, planning teams should define alternative futures and discuss them fully. Products of the environmental assessment may need to be revised or fine-tuned after completing this task.

Many excellent references offer approaches for developing alternative future scenarios. Among these, Paul J. H. Schoemaker (1995) recommends the following steps in scenario development:

- Define the scope
- Identify major stakeholders
- Identify basic trends
- Identify key uncertainties
- Construct initial scenario themes
- Check for consistency and plausibility
- Develop learning scenarios
- Identify research needs
- Develop quantitative models
- Evolve toward decision scenarios

This approach enables organizational leadership to consider and seriously analyze diverse alternative futures and distill a composite scenario (or scenarios) from this broad view of the future. It is important to consider that while a scenario exercise may have varying usefulness for management or planning staff, who consider potential futures on a regular basis, it can be a helpful tool for trustees or physicians who are not focused on specific market or sector trends. Exhibit 6.16 shows a scenario exercise that was used by the Strategic Planning Steering Committee at Yavapai Regional Medical Center (Arizona).

In contrast, most healthcare organizations typically rely—explicitly or implicitly—on the planning staff to develop a single future environmental scenario by extrapolating current trends and incorporating current hot issues.

Regardless of the approach used, the result should be an explicit set of underlying assumptions about the future, on which the remaining planning analyses and outputs will be based. Exhibit 6.17 presents an example of the results of this process.

As exhibit 6.17 illustrates, the assumptions should be stated briefly to avoid unnecessarily complicating the presentation of the future

Exhibit 6.16: Steering Committee Scenario Exercise: Shift to Value Payments for Yavapai Regional Medical Center (YRMC), 2015

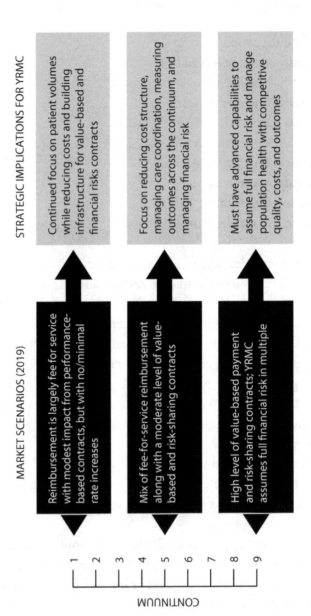

MARKET SCENARIOS (2019)

Reimbursement is largely fee for service with modest impact from performance-based contracts, but with no/minimal rate increases

Mix of fee-for-service reimbursement along with a moderate level of value-based and risk-sharing contracts

High level of value-based payment and risk-sharing contracts; YRMC assumes full financial risk in multiple

STRATEGIC IMPLICATIONS FOR YRMC

Continued focus on patient volumes while reducing costs and building infrastructure for value-based and financial risks contracts

Focus on reducing cost structure, managing care coordination, measuring outcomes across the continuum, and managing financial risk

Must have advanced capabilities to assume full financial risk and manage population health with competitive quality, costs, and outcomes

CONTINUUM
1
2
3
4
5
6
7
8
9

Each steering committee member selects where on the continuum she believes the market will evolve by 2019; the numeric rating drives a discussion of the "average score," interpreted as the most likely future scenario environment in which the organization will operate. This concise, simple summary of a potential future environment is a powerful guide by which to consider, or in many cases reconsider, critical planning issues and, subsequently, organizational mission and vision.

Identification of Critical Planning Issues

The final task in the environmental assessment is to determine what critical planning issues need to be resolved during the strategic

---

Exhibit 6.17: Future Assumptions Regarding the National and Local Market, Fiscal Year 2017 to Fiscal Year 2022

- Provider success will be based on delivering value, as defined by high-quality services at a low cost.
- Fee-for-service reimbursement will remain but will account for a lower percentage of most healthcare providers' revenue.
- Regional health systems will become more prevalent, with many markets consisting of only a few large systems.
- Consolidation in the provider and insurance market will give way to a focus on integration of recently partnered organizations.
- Primary care will play an increasingly central role in population health management.
- Nontraditional competitors will more frequently enter the healthcare market, with a focus on differentiating based on technology or customer service.
- Financial pressures will be exacerbated as commercial-payment increases slow to low single-digit levels and states manage budget issues.
- A significant proportion of physicians will be employed by hospitals, systems, or large multispecialty practices.
- Technological advances will continue to shift services to the outpatient setting.

© 2017 Veralon Partners Inc.

planning process. All of the preceding analysis feeds into this final result. The determination is subjective and usually evolves through an iterative process of some or all of the steps described in the next paragraph, depending on the size and complexity of the organization, the issues it faces, and the extent to which participative processes are used in strategic planning.

After the planning analyst or planning staff members select an initial list of issues, senior management team members review and revise the list, alone or together. The list may then go to the strategic planning committee members, individually or collectively, who will perform the same review. The issue list may then be accepted as a basis for moving forward or returned to the planning or senior management staff for further work. Exhibit 6.18 shows a worksheet used by a health system in Nevada to facilitate the prioritization of critical planning issues.

Typical critical planning issues that are common to strategic plans today are

- achieving sufficient scale and scope of services (via organic growth or affiliation),
- delivering and demonstrating value,
- constructing an effective and integrated delivery system,
- the need for significant improvement in financial performance,
- managing population health,
- developing clinical programs, and
- improving competitive positioning.

A variety of largely operational and quasi-strategic matters frequently emerge as critical issues in the environmental assessment. Leaders are often tempted to enumerate dozens of "important" issues that need to be resolved to ensure future success. But by doing so, they sacrifice strategic clarity and precision in the name of comprehensiveness and political expediency.

Exhibit 6.18: Critical Planning Issue Prioritization Worksheet, 2017

Instructions: Allocate 100 points among the emerging issues to indicate priority (more points = higher priority)

Emerging Issue	Description	Allocated Points
Integration	Seamlessly connect all aspects of the system operationally and electronically, with a focus on shared incentives and accountability	
Financial improvement	Stabilize and improve financial performance and position to ensure the system is able to fund both routine and strategic priorities moving forward	
Organizational design	Redesign the organizational structure, where necessary, to ensure the proper flow of information and decision making	
Culture transformation	Develop a consistent organization-wide culture based on a unique set of values that will make the system attractive to both customers and employees	
Physician alignment	Establish formal relationships with physicians across all specialties that are mutually beneficial and successful	
Service portfolio	Implement the ideal product and market mix to bolster and sustain long-term growth	
Population health management	Set mechanisms and processes to improve the health of a defined population(s) within the service area	
Partnerships	Affiliate with organizations and/or provider groups through a variety of models to extend the system's reach or grow in desired markets and services	
Value	Improve clinical outcomes and customer experience at the lowest possible cost	
	Total Points	100

Only a limited number of issues can and should be dealt with in the strategic planning process if the planning is to lead to a successful outcome. Exhibit 6.19 depicts how one healthcare delivery system subdivided the defined issues into two categories: critical strategic priorities and critical resource priorities. This approach is one reasonable way to handle an otherwise thorny political situation.

Few healthcare organizations have so many critical issues that they cannot be condensed into five to seven strategic issue categories. Increasingly, as planning horizons have condensed from five years or more years to three to five years because of increased sector uncertainty, some organizations are limiting their critical planning issues to as few as three key priorities. Failure to limit the number of issues to address in subsequent planning activities almost always dooms the strategic planning process. It is impossible to effectively tackle an excessive number of issues concurrently, and doing so may confuse organizational leadership about what issues are truly critical to strategic success.

Exhibit 6.19: One Healthcare System's Critical Issues Categorization, 2015

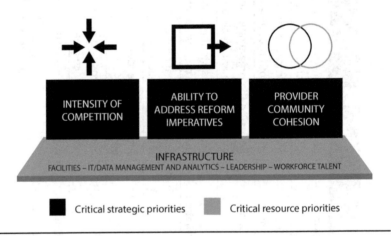

© 2017 Veralon Partners Inc.

CONCLUSION

A brief and high-level list of critical planning issues that require resolution is an excellent springboard to the next two planning activities: establishing overall or corporate direction and formulating core strategies. Such a list reduces voluminous data and other information collected during the environmental assessment to a manageable amount and energizes organizational leadership to move forward on strategic planning with a clear focus on issues of immense importance to the organization.

SUGGESTED READINGS

American Hospital Association. "AHA Environmental Scan." Published annually in the September issue of *H&HN*. www.hhnmag.com/articles/3199-american-hospital-association-environmental-scan.

American Hospital Association Resource Center blog. http://aharesourcecenter.wordpress.com.

Health Affairs. Published monthly. www.healthaffairs.org.

Healthcare Financial Management. Published monthly. www.hfma.org/hfm.

Journal of Healthcare Management. Published every other month. www.ache.org/pubs/journals.

Medicare Payment Advisory Commission. *Report to the Congress: Medicare Payment Policy.* Published annually in March. www.medpac.gov.

MGMA Connection. "The State of Medical Practice." Published annually in the January issue. www.mgma.com/store/magazines.

Modern Healthcare. "Healthcare Business and Policy Outlook." Published annually in the first issue of the year. www.modern-healthcare.com.

Society for Healthcare Strategy & Market Development and Health
Administration Press. *Futurescan: Healthcare Trends and Implications*. Published annually. http://shsmd.org/futurescan.

REFERENCES

Hamel, G., and C. K. Prahalad. 1994. "Competing for the Future."
Harvard Business Review 72 (4): 122–28.
Schoemaker, P. J. H. 1995. "Scenario Planning: A Tool for Strategic
Thinking." *Sloan Management Review* 36 (2): 25–41.

CHAPTER 7

Phase 2: Organizational Direction

If you do not change direction, you may end up where you are heading.

—*Lao Tzu (attributed)*

When it comes to the future, there are three kinds of people: those who let it happen, those who make it happen, and those who wonder what happened.

—*John M. Richardson Jr.*

Good business leaders create a vision, articulate the vision, passionately own the vision, and relentlessly drive it to completion.

—*Jack Welch*

The second activity of the strategic planning process, establishing the organizational direction, initiates in earnest the process of looking forward to chart what the organization's future might be. This activity sets direction at a high level, encompassing mission, vision, overall organizational strategy, and values. Subsequent activities address important components of future direction and the particular aspects of implementation. Exhibit 7.1 provides a context for the principal outputs of the organizational direction activity.

Exhibit 7.1: Organizational Direction

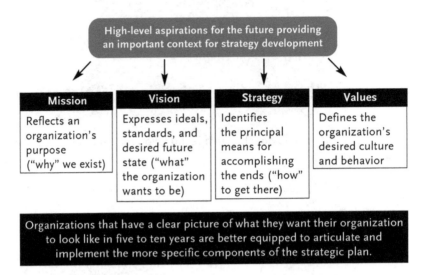

High-level aspirations for the future providing an important context for strategy development

Mission	Vision	Strategy	Values
Reflects an organization's purpose ("why" we exist)	Expresses ideals, standards, and desired future state ("what" the organization wants to be)	Identifies the principal means for accomplishing the ends ("how" to get there)	Defines the organization's desired culture and behavior

Organizations that have a clear picture of what they want their organization to look like in five to ten years are better equipped to articulate and implement the more specific components of the strategic plan.

© 2017 Veralon Partners Inc.

REVIEW OF THE LITERATURE

The strategic planning literature highlights the importance of a clear mission and vision to the organization's future success. Peter M. Ginter, W. Jack Duncan, and Linda E. Swayne (2013) note that mission, vision, values, and strategic goals are accurately called directional strategies because they guide strategists in making key organizational decisions. Russ Coile Jr. (1994) describes the interrelationship between vision and strategy as an arrow-to-target process. A shared vision is the target, and strategic planning is the arrow. Timothy R. Clark (2011) writes that organizational vision has three operational functions: a cognitive function to educate, an emotional function to motivate, and an organizational function to coordinate. When all three functions are in place and actively applied, the vision guides the answers to thousands of operational questions and leads to coordinated, effective, and efficient action.

There are, however, caveats to developing mission and vision statements. Christopher K. Bart (2002, 41) writes, "For many senior executives, mission statements don't seem to be worth the paper on which they are written. They don't seem to be of any value." Nonetheless, he goes on to say, "Surprisingly, mission statements (and their accompanying vision and values proclamations) continue to be considered one of the most popular management tools in the world and have even been ranked at least in the top two practices in global usage by Bain & Company since 1993."

As Bart suggests and as the authors' experiences confirm, the reason for the popularity and prevalence of mission and vision statements is that they make a promise and focus the organization's activities on fulfilling it. Most often, healthcare organizations that clearly express their basic purpose in a mission statement and paint an accurate picture of what they want their organization to look like in five to ten years in a vision statement stand a good chance of articulating and implementing the specific components of the strategic plan, thereby realizing that vision. Failure to specify a mission that is compelling and unique to the healthcare organization, or to define a clear and exciting vision, hinders attempts to resolve strategic issues and to make progress toward a better future.

Robert S. Kaplan, David P. Norton, and Edward A. Barrows Jr. (2008) note that if vision statements are to guide strategy development, they must be inspirational, aspirational, and measurable. To be useful, a statement should also provide a clear focus for the strategy by including a measurable outcome and a distinct target. Kaplan, Norton, and Barrows suggest that a well-crafted vision statement should include three components: a quantified success indicator, a definition of a niche, and a time line. These three components are evident in the example from Leeds University in the United Kingdom (Kaplan, Norton, and Barrows 2008, 4): "By 2015 (*timeline*), our distinctive ability to integrate world-class research, scholarship, and education (*niche*) will have secured us a place among the top 50 universities in the world (*quantifiable success indicator*)."

Michael E. Porter (1996, 62) cautions that all too frequently in US industry, "bit by bit, almost imperceptibly, management tools have taken the place of strategy. As managers push to improve on all fronts, they move farther away from viable competitive positions." By failing to focus on what will distinguish their organizations in the future, and thus on the essence of effective organizational direction, these companies have difficulty translating gains in operational improvements into sustained profitability.

GUIDELINES FOR DEVELOPING AN EFFECTIVE ORGANIZATIONAL DIRECTION

While specifying direction is necessary and important, developing effective organizational direction statements is a monumental challenge, especially in healthcare organizations. Common problems in direction statements include extreme wordiness; confusion of mission, vision, strategy, and values and a mixture of some in each statement; redundancy among statements; lack of precision; and failure to be farsighted.

Effective statements must be, above all, meaningful, motivational, and memorable. For example, The Joint Commission expects leadership *and* rank-and-file employees in the healthcare organizations it reviews to know their mission statements. But how many mission statements are clear and succinct enough that the organization's employees can readily state it?

Exhibit 7.2 provides a summary of the guidelines for successfully navigating this activity of the strategic planning process. Key points include the following:

- *Sharp, tailored, directional statements are most useful.* These statements should be highly focused and specific to the particular organization that created them; platitudes and verbosity have no place here.

Exhibit 7.2: Developing the Plan: Organizational Direction

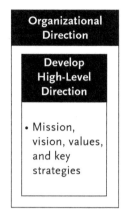

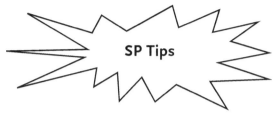

Organizational Direction
Develop High-Level Direction
• Mission, vision, values, and key strategies

SP Tips

- Develop sharp, tailored, directional statements
- Establish one vision, one direction
  - In large organizations, operating unit direction *must* be consistent with corporate direction
- This is the most important corporate or systemwide strategic planning activity

© 2017 Veralon Partners Inc.

- *For any complex, multientity organization, one vision and one direction are essential.* Successful organizations have a unified direction that is relevant to every entity within them. Establishing an organizational direction at every subsidiary would not only be cumbersome for the strategic planning process, it would also likely lead to inconsistent or conflicting strategies. All subsidiaries must move in the same direction; major, and sometimes minor, differences in vision and direction are divisive and potentially destructive.

- *Organizational direction is the most critical part of the board's and CEO's contribution to strategic planning.* It must emanate from and be fully supported by all elements of corporate or system leadership.

If planning for the future position of the organization starts with poorly conceived, uncertain, or confusing directional statements, the planning process may eventually derail. Getting it back on track will be difficult, if not impossible. Beginning with clear organizational direction, on the other hand, helps focus the subsequent detailed strategy-formulation and implementation-planning activities, making it critical to strategic planning success. The organizational direction statements generally fall into two categories: legacy statements (mission and values) and core strategy statements (vision and organization strategy).

Organizations typically have long-standing mission and values statements. A strategic planning process is an opportune time to reflect on these statements and consider whether the mission still represents the reasons the organization exists and whether the values still represent the organization's desired culture and behavior. It is common for these statements to remain wholly unchanged or only slightly modified as a result of this examination. While many of the problems of organizational direction statements referenced earlier may apply to an organization's current mission or values, the two most common reasons for revising these statements are as follows:

- *The mission and values are not concise or clear.* While it is helpful for employees to have knowledge of an organization's future direction via a vision statement, it is essential that all employees know and understand the organization's mission and values, particularly the latter, as these represent how an employee should function on a day-to-day basis. A simple litmus test is to consider if the mission and values statements can easily be recited by employees at all levels of the organization. If not, then these statements likely need to be reconsidered. This situation does not necessarily indicate the essence of those statements needs to change—simply that the way they are stated can be improved.
- *The mission and values do not reflect significant changes in the organization.* The incremental changes most healthcare organizations experience from year to year do not represent a significant divergence from their mission or values. However, if an organization enters an entirely

new business or exits an existing business, the fundamental purpose or culture of the organization may change. Similarly, if an organization has a major growth spurt (these days, often the result of inorganic growth) or merges with another organization, these legacy statements may not be applicable.

The following sections outline some things to consider in the event that the mission or values statements require reexamination.

DEVELOPMENT OF THE MISSION STATEMENT

Mission statements should be relatively timeless in the absence of significant organizational change. Some organizations' current statements will not require alterations as part of the strategic planning process. However, if reexamination and retooling of the mission statement are called for, the starting point should be the current statement.

Mission Statement Characteristics

Effective mission statements are brief and fundamental statements of organizational purpose. A mission statement should clearly communicate to the board, employees, and other internal and external constituencies why the organization exists and what important purpose it intends to achieve. Influential management consultant, writer, and professor Peter Drucker is reputed to have said that the content of a mission statement should be small enough to fit on a T-shirt. Also, mission statements commonly stray into strategy, which should be avoided. If a mission statement addresses "how" an organization will proceed or act, it should be reconsidered.

Exhibit 7.3 presents several examples of recently developed mission statements for healthcare organizations, as well as examples from major companies outside the healthcare field. Note the precision, clarity, and brevity of the nonhealthcare mission statements compared with even these exceptional examples of healthcare mission statements. Interesting, too, is how 3M, GE, Nike, and Google capture the essence of their purpose without resorting to descriptions of the business, products, or markets. These statements should inspire healthcare leaders to think carefully and creatively about the true purpose of their organizations.

Mission Statement Development Process

The mission statement development process varies by organization, but in any organization, significant input is the board's most fundamental contribution to organization policy and strategic direction. Development begins with the strategic planning committee, which

Exhibit 7.3: Mission Statement Examples

Nonhealthcare
GE: To invent the next industrial era, to build, move, power, and cure the world.
Google: To organize the world's information and make it universally accessible and useful.
Nike: To bring inspiration and innovation to every athlete in the world.
3M: To solve unsolved problems innovatively.
Healthcare
Banner Health (Phoenix, AZ): We exist to make a difference in people's lives through patient care.
Jefferson Health (Philadelphia, PA): Health is all we do.
Randolph Hospital (Asheboro, NC): To provide quality healthcare and foster health and wellness in our communities.

may hold two to three sessions at least partly devoted to a discussion of mission. These sessions typically encompass

- scenario development and generation of a composite future scenario (as discussed in chapter 6),
- review of the definition of a mission statement and examination of the current statement,
- review of other healthcare organizations' mission statements (and possibly some nonhealthcare mission statements), and
- review and modification of a new draft mission statement.

Strategic planning committee or board members should not be wordsmiths for the proposed mission statement. They should instead concentrate on what the mission statement is trying to convey, focusing on substantive changes in content. A group discussion is not the place to rewrite, in whole or in part, the mission statement, as it is a cumbersome, tedious, and ultimately unproductive approach. Drafting or redrafting the document should be left to an individual or a small group once the discussion sessions have yielded the statement's focus.

DEVELOPMENT OF THE VALUES STATEMENT

Like the mission statement, the values statement is widely disseminated to internal and external constituencies. In the absence of significant organizational or environmental changes, this statement is relatively timeless and may not require major modification.

With the proliferation of mergers and other forms of affiliation; the growth of integrated delivery systems; and, for some, disaffiliation and disintegration, few healthcare organizations have been untouched by the waves of change sweeping the field. In these new, larger organizations, diverse cultures are brought together, and existing values are blended into, or in some cases imposed on, the new entity. The core of the values statement is a representation of the desired character of the new organizational culture and sets forth the manner in which that character is conveyed to employees and other stakeholders. As some organizations downsize, restructure, and divest themselves of component parts, the values of the surviving entities often must be reexamined.

In stable, successful healthcare organizations, a values statement can be gleaned from organizational behavior. Observance of the day-to-day practices of the employees and of board policy and performance will lead to a fairly clear picture of the organization's values. This values statement can be fine-tuned by leadership to reflect some minor modification of organizational behavior and then serve as the product of the values definition task.

For other healthcare organizations (e.g., brand-new organizations, those with high organic growth, those in rapid organic decline), a values statement should be developed through a top-down process similar to that recommended for the mission statement. Where current organizational values are determined to be inadequate or not conducive to providing high-quality healthcare and new or significantly different organizational values must be instituted, leadership must discover how the existing values came into being. Then the organization must conduct a self-examination to create a new values statement for the future.

Examples of values statements from two health systems, typical of what many healthcare organizations aspire to, are illustrated in exhibit 7.4. Note, as well, the Disney Corporation and Mercedes-Benz USA values statements, and given the general public knowledge of these organizations, how tailored and descriptive a values statement can be.

The vision statement and the organization strategy statement represent core strategy elements and, unlike the mission and values, should be developed anew in virtually every strategic planning process. These statements progress beyond why the organization exists and describe what the organization wants to be and how the organization will get there.

Exhibit 7.4: Values Statement Examples

Nonhealthcare
Disney Corporation
• No cynicism
• Nurturing and promulgation of wholesome American values
• Creativity, dreams, and imagination
• Fanatical attention to consistency and detail
• Preservation and control of the Disney image
Mercedes-Benz USA
• The audacity to reject compromise
• The instinct to protect what matters
• The commitment to honor legacy
• The vision to consider every detail
• The foresight to take responsibility
• The integrity to outperform expectations
Healthcare
Memorial Health System (Springfield, IL)
• Community responsibility
• Equal access
• Excellence in performance
• Integrity in relationships
• Respect for the individual
• Service to humanity
• Value of employees
Banner Health (Phoenix, AZ)
• Excellence
• People above all
• Results

DEVELOPMENT OF THE VISION STATEMENT

Planning teams should consider vision statements and mission statements simultaneously, and the development of the two should follow the same process and general principles. The main distinction between mission statements and vision statements is that mission is about purpose ("Why does the organization exist?") and vision is about the future ("What does an organization want to be?"). In addition, mission statements are not time limited, whereas vision statements refer to a particular future point or period and generally must be updated and revised with each complete strategic planning process.

Vision Statement Characteristics

Unlike the mission statement, the current vision statement likely requires substantial change if it is to be an effective guide for the organization's future direction. But many vision statements share two main problems with mission statements—cumbersome length and inappropriate inclusion of strategy.

Effective vision statements conform to the guidelines listed in exhibit 7.1. The vision statement should be a vehicle by which to communicate a preferred future state of the organization to internal constituencies. Historically, organizations have considered vision statements as far as ten years and beyond into the future. However, given the rapid change in the healthcare field—recently and possibly for the foreseeable future—many healthcare organizations are limiting their vision statements to five to ten years. The statement should be aspirational given current circumstances and conditions, and it should represent such an exciting and desirable state of being that it motivates and energizes all elements of the organization through the ground-level strategies and actions that support it. Exhibit 7.5 shows concepts that frequently appear in vision statements of various types of healthcare organizations.

The vision statement should project far enough into the future that the point of unpredictability is reached. This extended time frame should encourage organizational leaders to be imaginative in their views of the future characteristics of the organization while avoiding the urge to analyze their way into the future.

Exhibit 7.5: Vision Statement Concepts

Organization Type	Common Vision Concepts
Community hospital	• Improve patient/customer experience • Provide best value in healthcare services • Become a preferred physician partner
Academic medical center	• Innovate • Become a research or education leader • Provide world-class care
Integrated health system	• Transform healthcare delivery • Improve population health • Be a leading community partner
Post-acute provider	• Shift the care setting to home • Improve quality of life
Insurer	• Reduce healthcare costs • Improve the total healthcare experience • Provide access to care for broad populations

© 2017 Veralon Partners Inc.

Several examples of healthcare organization vision statements that conform to this description are presented in exhibit 7.6, along with a few classic and contemporary examples from major corporations outside the healthcare field.

Here, as with the mission statement examples, the precision, clarity, and brevity of the nonhealthcare examples are striking. Those examples also illustrate the recommended vision principles—stretching, motivating, and inspiring the organizations to achieve what nearly all experts would have deemed improbable, if not impossible, at the time they were developed. Healthcare organizations are making progress in vision development, and the examples in exhibit 7.6 illustrate this effort.

Exhibit 7.6: Vision Statement Examples

Nonhealthcare (Historical)
Ford (early 1900s): Democratize the automobile
Honda (1970s): We will destroy Yamaha
Sony (early 1950s): Become the company most known for changing the worldwide poor-quality image of Japanese products
Stanford University (1940s): Become the Harvard of the west

Nonhealthcare (Contemporary)
Amazon: Our vision is to be Earth's most customer centric company
Boeing: People working together as a global enterprise for aerospace industry leadership
Google: Provide access to the world's information in one click

Healthcare (Contemporary)
Banner Health (Phoenix, AZ): We will be a national leader recognized for clinical excellence and innovation, preferred for a highly coordinated patient experience, and distinguished by the quality of our people.
Jefferson Health (Philadelphia, PA): We will reimagine health, health education, and discovery to create unparalleled value and to be the most trusted healthcare partner.
Randolph Hospital (Asheboro, NC): The preferred provider for high quality care, creating better health in our communities and recognized for excellence in all that we do.

The strategic plan of Banner Health provides an example of the power of a bold organizational vision. In 2000, Banner was struggling financially and organizationally after the merger of two disparate health systems. Banner Health aspired to be in the top tier of medical centers nationally but recognized that given its current situation,

Exhibit 7.7: Banner Health's 20-Year Vision

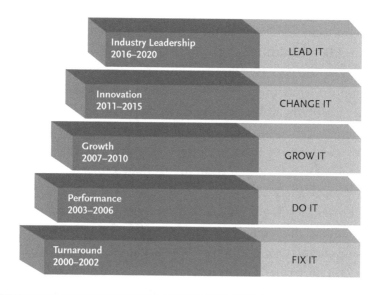

Industry Leadership 2016–2020	LEAD IT
Innovation 2011–2015	CHANGE IT
Growth 2007–2010	GROW IT
Performance 2003–2006	DO IT
Turnaround 2000–2002	FIX IT

this vision could be a 20-year journey (see exhibit 7.7). Banner set its long-range vision and also established interim targets (Compass Clinical Consulting 2011). The organization is largely living up to the vision it set in 2000—an impressive feat.

Vision Statement Development Process

The suggestions discussed earlier related to the mission statement apply to the development of a vision statement, too. Interactions among the board, strategic planning committee, and other key leaders should produce an effective vision statement without excessive attention to wordsmithery.

DEVELOPMENT OF OVERALL
ORGANIZATION STRATEGY

The mission and vision address the why and what of future direction. Many healthcare organizations cannot or do not distinguish between the why or what and the how of future direction and inappropriately include strategy in mission or vision statements. They have difficulty determining a principal means (i.e., strategy) to accomplish the articulated ends (i.e., mission and vision) from those ends. Such an organization often sets forth multiple and diverse overall strategies, which compounds the confusion and results in no strategy at all.

Porter (1996, 78) argues that many senior managers mistake operational effectiveness for strategy and as a result move away from viable competitive positions: "Improving operational effectiveness is a necessary part of management, but it is not strategy. In confusing the two, managers have unintentionally backed into a way of thinking about competition that is driving many industries toward competitive convergence, which is in no one's best interest and is not inevitable." The result: Overall organization strategy is often the least clearly defined element of future direction.

Strategy Development Frameworks

Raymond E. Miles and Charles C. Snow (1978) developed a typology to describe a hospital's strategic orientation, classifying hospitals into four categories: prospectors, defenders, analyzers, and reactors.

- A *prospector* is an organization that makes frequent changes in and additions to its services and markets; it consistently responds rapidly to market opportunities by being the first to provide a new service or develop a new market.

- A *defender* offers a fairly stable set of services to defined markets and tends to ignore changes that do not directly affect current operations, focusing instead on doing its best in the current arena.
- An *analyzer*, like a defender, maintains a relatively stable base of services but selectively develops new services or markets the way the prospector does. However, the analyzer rarely is the first to provide new services or expand into new markets, choosing instead to monitor actions of others and follow with a well thought out, thorough approach.
- A *reactor* is an organization that does not appear to respond consistently to changes in the market and seems to lack a coherent strategy. The reactor may, on occasion, be an early entrant into a new market or service but usually is forced into action by external events or after considerable evidence of potential for success.

A healthcare organization may have difficulty articulating its strategy as that of a defender, an analyzer, or a reactor. As Stephen M. Shortell, Ellen M. Morrison, and Bernard Friedman (1989) point out, many healthcare organizations espouse a prospector strategy, but few truly follow it, which may partly explain their confusion about overall strategy.

Another framework for overall strategy that is prevalent in general business, developed by Porter (1980), suggests that companies follow one of three principal strategies (singly or in combination) to create a defendable position: overall cost leadership, differentiation, or focus (also called niching).

The overall cost leadership strategy is achieved through a set of aggressive policies that ensure construction of efficient facilities, continuous pursuit of cost reduction, and systematic control of costs and overhead. Differentiation of a product or service offering means creating something that is perceived throughout the field as unique. The differentiation strategy does not ignore costs, but they are not the primary strategic focus. The focus strategy centers on a particular buyer or geographic market. While low-cost and differentiation strategies aim to establish the organization as a leader across the field, the focus strategy aims to serve a particular target well, and policies are developed with this in mind. The organization is then able to serve its narrow target focus more effectively than those competing broadly.

Organization Strategy Characteristics

Gary Hamel (1996, 70) argues that successful strategy must be revolutionary: "Never has the world been more hospitable to industry revolutionaries and more hostile to industry incumbents." Hamel describes nine routes to industry revolution that involve reconceiving a product or service, redefining market space, and redrawing industry boundaries.

Regardless of which strategy framework it adopts, the organization must choose from among available alternative future strategies to have a high probability of realizing its vision. A principal strategy needs to be selected and articulated to all affected internal organizational constituencies as a key part of the organization's direction.

Exhibit 7.8 presents several examples of strategy statements from organizations inside and outside healthcare—all of them providing clear, discernable summaries of the organizations' strategic intentions. Such statements, however, are difficult to find because so few organizations, especially not-for-profits, pursue any discernible strategy. Many are still on the rebound from the trendy strategy of the 1990s, integration, and of the first decade of the twenty-first century, refocusing on the core business. Opportunism, or in Miles and Snow's (1978) typology, being an analyzer or a reactor,

Exhibit 7.8: Strategy Statement Examples

Nonhealthcare
Nordstrom: Service to the customer
Procter & Gamble: Product excellence

Healthcare
Anthem • Create the best health care value in our industry • Excel at day-to-day execution • Capitalize on new opportunities to drive growth
Ascension Health (St. Louis, MO): We will fulfill our promise to those we serve by delivering Healthcare That Works, Healthcare That Is Safe, and Healthcare That Leaves No One Behind, for Life.
Banner Health (Phoenix, AZ) • Be recognized for clinical excellence and innovation • Develop a highly coordinated patient experience • Be distinguished by the quality of our people
Community Health Systems (Brentwood, TN): Effectively integrating organizations and improving hospital operations

rather than a clearly defined proactive strategy, seems to be the norm today.

Organization Strategy Development Process

The process of developing overall organization strategy is similar to that described earlier for the mission and vision statements. However, compared to the mission and vision statements, the strategy statement emanates to a greater degree from planning staff and top management versus the strategic planning committee and the board.

CONCLUSION

Organizational direction produces four critical outputs—mission, vision, strategy, and values statements—that are developed during phase 2 of the strategic planning process. With direction identified, productive movement into the next level of detail in strategic planning—strategy formulation (made up of major initiatives, goals, and objectives) to address the important issues outlined in phase 1—may begin.

As the organization moves further into the how of strategic planning, the roles and responsibilities of management expand. The board, both directly and through its strategic planning committee, may have had significant input into the organizational direction because it represents the major policy elements of the strategic plan; with the completion of the organizational direction activities, the transition from board-driven strategic planning to staff-driven strategic planning begins.

REFERENCES

Bart, C. K. 2002. "Creating Effective Mission Statements: Recapturing the Power and Glory of Mission Is Possible with Careful Planning and Implementation." *Health Progress* 83 (5): 41–55.

Clark, T. R. 2011. "The Power of Vision Provides Organizations with Direction, Inspiration." *Deseret News*. Published February 14. www.deseretnews.com/article/705366518/The-power-of-vision-provides-organizations-with-direction-inspiration.html.

Coile, R. C., Jr. 1994. "Making Strategic Planning a Vision-Driven Process." *Hospital Strategy Report* 6 (10): 8.8.

Compass Clinical Consulting. 2011. "A Fine Choice." Published March 11. www.compass-clinical.com/wp-content/uploads/2013/10/fine-monograph3.pdf.

Ginter, P. M., W. J. Duncan, and L. E. Swayne. 2013. *Strategic Management of Health Care Organizations*, 7th ed. San Francisco: Jossey-Bass.

Hamel, G. 1996. "Strategy as Revolution." *Harvard Business Review*, July–August, 69–82.

Kaplan, R. S., D. P. Norton, and E. A. Barrows Jr. 2008. *Developing the Strategy: Vision, Value Gaps, and Analysis.* Boston: Harvard Business School Publishing.

Miles, R. E., and C. C. Snow. 1978. *Organizational Strategy, Structure, and Process.* New York: McGraw-Hill.

Porter, M. E. 1996. "What Is Strategy?" *Harvard Business Review*, November–December, 61–78.

———. 1980. *Competitive Strategy.* New York: Free Press.

Shortell, S. M., E. M. Morrison, and B. Friedman. 1989. *Strategic Choices for America's Hospitals.* New York: Wiley.

CHAPTER 8

Phase 3: Strategy Formulation

> The only constant in our business is that everything is changing. We have to take advantage of change and not let it take advantage of us. We have to be ahead of the game.
>
> —*Michael Dell (attributed)*

> Sound strategy starts with having the right goal.
>
> —*Michael Porter*

FROM VISION TO GOALS

Once leaders have defined the overall direction of their organization, they can turn to determining its goals, objectives, and future strategic development. As emphasized in chapter 7, significant progress must be made in a number of key areas to achieve the vision of the next five to ten years. Exhibit 8.1 shows the critical relationship between organizational direction and strategy formulation and defines the outputs of each strategic planning activity.

Exhibit 8.2 highlights a few especially important points about the strategy formulation phase of strategic planning. Broadening the number and type of internal participants involved in plan development and bringing multiple diverse perspectives to bear on strategy formulation will increase the probability of success. In large, multi-entity organizations, the strategy formulation framework usually begins at the system or corporate level and cascades down to the operating units for their respective strategy formulations.

Exhibit 8.1: From Organizational Direction to Strategy Formulation

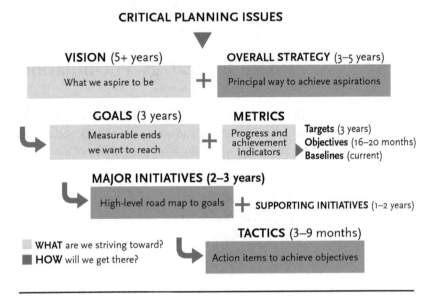

CRITICAL PLANNING ISSUES

VISION (5+ years)

What we aspire to be

+

OVERALL STRATEGY (3–5 years)

Principal way to achieve aspirations

GOALS (3 years)

Measurable ends we want to reach

+

METRICS

Progress and achievement indicators

▶ **Targets** (3 years)
Objectives (16–20 months)
Baselines (current)

MAJOR INITIATIVES (2–3 years)

High-level road map to goals **+** SUPPORTING INITIATIVES (1–2 years)

TACTICS (3–9 months)

▪ **WHAT** are we striving toward?
▪ **HOW** will we get there?

Action items to achieve objectives

© 2017 Veralon Partners Inc.

For many organizations, the most difficult part of strategic planning is moving from the vision to the next level of detail: the goals. Identifying hundreds of goals that support the vision is tempting but should be avoided, as it results in an unwieldy plan that cannot be implemented. Healthcare organizations also struggle with setting measurable, clear goals, tending instead to specify a series of activities or processes or a vague directional intent (e.g., "improve quality"). This chapter addresses these problems directly.

Strategic planning is, in essence, the process of making difficult choices among competing priorities and focusing the organization's limited resources on the areas that will yield the greatest payoff. For strategic planning to be effective, that focus must be maintained throughout the process—and especially in the transition from vision to goals. Successful organizations identify only a small set of goals

Exhibit 8.2: Developing the Plan: Strategy Formulation

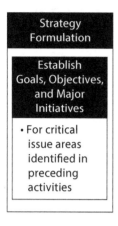

Strategy
Formulation

Establish
Goals, Objectives,
and Major
Initiatives

- For critical
  issue areas
  identified in
  preceding
  activities

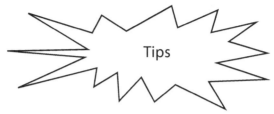

Tips

- This is an excellent time or phase to get broad
  involvement of internal constituents
- Overall corporate or system goals direct operating
  unit goals and objectives
- To be effective, the strategy needs to address a
  limited number (no more than ten and preferably
  no more than five) of the most critical issues

© 2017 Veralon Partners Inc.

that are imperatives for realizing the vision—preferably no more than five, and certainly no more than ten.

Moving from vision to goals is most readily accomplished through a three-phase process:

1. Determine or affirm critical issues
2. Formulate strategic options and recommendations
3. Identify goals

Determining Critical Issues

Critical issues are determined by examining the organization's mission, vision, and key organizational strategy in light of the initial critical planning issues defined in the environmental assessment (see exhibit 8.3). Often the critical planning issues the organization defined in phase 1 survive largely intact as the final set of critical issues. Sometimes the issues may need to be reshaped because of conclusions reached in the organizational direction phase.

Exhibit 8.3: The Strategy Formulation Process

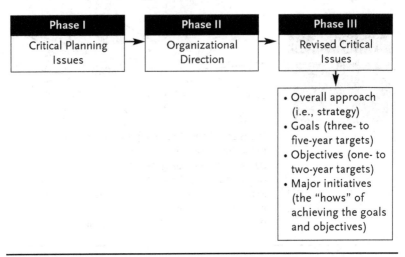

Phase I	Phase II	Phase III
Critical Planning Issues	Organizational Direction	Revised Critical Issues

- Overall approach (i.e., strategy)
- Goals (three- to five-year targets)
- Objectives (one- to two-year targets)
- Major initiatives (the "hows" of achieving the goals and objectives)

Determining what constitutes a critical issue is clearly subjective, and healthcare executives are commonly confused by this step. Typically, critical issues stand out as central to achieving the vision, have a deep potential impact on the organization, and cannot be addressed easily or resolved in the short term. Another commonly made distinction is that these issues deal primarily with concerns outside the realm of day-to-day operations.

One of two approaches is typically used to determine the final list of critical issues. The more process-intensive approach, used most often when the initial list of issues is large or controversial, consists of three steps. First, each member of the strategic planning committee identifies the top three or so issues, and they compile a master list. Assuming the priorities are not obvious from this first step, a second step is to have some discussion of what each issue is and why it is important. Some issues may fall off the list or be consolidated as a result. Third, the committee members are asked to vote for the top three issues; the most frequently named issues make the final list.

The second approach is for planning staff or a small group of members of senior management to narrow the number of potential issues down to no more than ten and present the findings of its analyses to the strategic planning committee for review and modification. It is important to specify why the selected areas are strategically significant and why other areas are not. Two representative lists of critical issues that resulted from such a process are shown in exhibit 8.4.

Preparing Strategic Options and Recommendations

Once critical issues are identified, the focus moves from issues to goals. A process-intensive approach is most likely to identify the best goals, objectives, major initiatives, and actions and to build support for plan implementation and action. The more process-intensive the approach, the more time required to complete it. A highly intensive approach can take as long as two or three months, while the least intensive approach can be completed in as few as three or four weeks. If the time frame for planning is a concern, the planning team should carefully consider the approach selected for this activity.

Exhibit 8.4: Critical Issues

Stony Brook Medicine (academic health system)	St. Mary's Health (community hospital)
• Network growth • System integration • Value	• Physician and provider partnerships • Coverage and distribution • Signature programs • Value for all stakeholders

Sources: Stony Brook Medicine (2016); St. Mary's Health (2015). Used with permission.

Leaders can choose from three basic paths to transition to goal setting:

1. *Move directly from critical issues to goals.* Planning staff, senior management, or the strategic planning committee (with assistance from the previous two constituencies) develop the goals without further analysis or process.

2. *Prepare strategic options and recommendations.* Preparing in-depth reports that consider strategic options can help to distinguish and prioritize alternatives. Planning staff prepare supporting documentation on each issue and recommend goals for review and modification by senior management and the strategic planning committee.

3. *Convene task forces to prepare strategic options and recommendations.* This option is similar to option 2, except that a multidisciplinary group of organizational representatives convenes for a limited period to assist in preparing the supporting documentation.

   The task force alternative has an additional benefit: It exposes important organizational stakeholders to the outline of the emerging strategic plan and constructively engages them in further definition of organizational strategy in areas that are personally significant and relevant. A few guidelines, presented in the following paragraphs, can help organizations to manage this third path.

Assemble the Task Force with Care

No foolproof formula exists for assembling task forces, but recognizing all the ends the organization is trying to accomplish and the potential incompatibility of those ends is a good starting point. A typical set of principles for task force composition includes the following:

- Gain broad representation from potentially affected constituencies
- Include enough diversity so that the task force is not biased toward any single perspective
- Achieve relatively good chemistry among the members
- Keep the group small enough that it is not unwieldy
- Select members who are interested enough to participate actively
- Choose a leader who will lead but not dominate

The task forces typically will meet three to four times over a period ranging from six to eight weeks (or longer). The members should understand and appreciate that their task is time limited and that they are not making decisions, only presenting alternatives and making recommendations to the strategic planning committee.

Give Task Force Guidelines and Support

Although active participation and free-flowing discussion are to be encouraged, some structure and staff support are necessary to achieve sound output and leave the participants feeling that they were constructively involved in the process. Expectations of the task forces need to be defined clearly at the outset, including the time frame for deliberation, questions to answer or issues to address, and likely structure of the output needed. Exhibits 8.5 and 8.6 give samples of guidance that might be provided to task forces. Appendix 8.1 presents an example of a full set of strategic options and recommendations developed using this outline. The planning team should assemble data and other relevant information collected in earlier planning activities and provide them to task force members before their first meeting. The planning staff should be introduced as staff support to the task forces and play a major role in logistical support, data support, and production of the strategic options and recommendations.

Exhibit 8.5: Task Force Overview: ABC Health System

Strategic Issue	Issues to Be Explored	Proposed Leadership and Membership Profile

1. Primary care network	• Size and distribution of the network
	• Operational and financial expectations
	• Mechanisms for incorporating physicians and extenders into the network
		• Leader: Primary care physician
		• Members:
		  – Managed care
		  – Marketing
		  – Senior management
		  – Nurse practitioners
		  – Practice managers

2. Cost position	• Cost target required to compete successfully
	• Schedule to attain targeted costs
	• Approaches to cost management and reduction
		• Leader: Chief financial officer
		• Members:
		  – Department chairs
		  – Senior management

3. Medical education	• Role of medical education in system
	• Expectations of medical education and criteria for evaluating residencies
	• Need for an academic affiliation
		• Leader: Teaching physician
		• Members:
		  – Physicians trained at system programs
		  – Other physicians
		  – Senior management

© 2017 Veralon Partners Inc.

Exhibit 8.6: Outline: Critical Issue Strategic Options and Recommendations

- Issue definition
- Background (including importance of resolving the issue)
- Strategies being employed by others faced with similar situations
- Options available, pros and cons, evaluation of options
- Recommended option(s) to pursue
- Major goals for a three- to five-year planning horizon; objectives for next year (or two); major initiatives (categories of activities) to achieve goals and objectives
- Barriers and constraints to achieving goals and objectives

© 2017 Veralon Partners Inc.

Identifying Goals

Ideally, the strategic options and recommendations will thoroughly review all aspects of the critical issue they address and present recommendations that allow a goal—or, occasionally, multiple goals—to be readily identified. It is the strategic planning committee's job to select a goal that will constructively and creatively deal with the critical issue and contribute to achieving part of the vision.

Typically, each task force leader presents the team's report to the strategic planning committee for review, modification, and, ultimately, acceptance. A goal is then identified, discussed, and modified before strategic planning committee approval. Exhibits 8.7 and 8.8 show the relationship between critical issues and goals.

Goals should be stated in measurable forms, whenever possible, and as targets for the future. However, this approach is not always practical or possible. The Regional Health System example shows goals that are described as qualitative future positions rather than quantitative endpoints. In such cases, it is important to define metrics related to the goals that can be monitored as a measurement of progress. Exhibit 8.9 provides an example of such metrics. Goals and objectives should be framed as ends to be achieved on the

Exhibit 8.7: Current and Desired Future State: Regional Health System

Critical Issue: Coordinate care to deliver value	
Current State (2017)	**Desired Future State (2022)**
Care across the health system is siloed or fragmented	Care is coordinated across the health system
View that customer = patient	View that customer = health partners (e.g., patients, community members, physicians, organizations)
Operates in a volume-driven fee-for-service environment	"Value plus volume" approach
Ability to take risk is limited	Able to take on risk for the entire population; impact on overall population health is significant
Critical Issue: Expand partnerships	
Current State (2017)	**Desired Future State (2022)**
Few alignment options to promote partnerships with physicians and other providers	Various strategies to align or partner with physicians and other providers are defined and implemented
Historical tendency to be an insular organization	Develop and strengthen partnerships to improve the health of the community
Increasingly challenging to recruit staff	Employer of choice that attracts staff locally, regionally, and nationally
Critical Issue: Grow across the full continuum of care	
Current State (2017)	**Desired Future State (2022)**
Focus on traditional acute care services and programs	Service portfolio appropriately meets the needs of the community through internal services or partnerships

(continued)

(continued from previous page)

Geographic reach extends beyond the primary service area, but focus tends to be local	Geographic focus extends beyond the primary service area to include a variety of populations throughout the region
Ad hoc approach to innovation	Innovative solutions are encouraged and routinely executed and embraced throughout the health system

© 2017 Veralon Partners Inc.

Exhibit 8.8: Critical Issues and Goals: Regional Health System

Critical Issues	Fiscal Year 2017–Fiscal Year 2022 Goals
Coordinate care to deliver value	Deliver high-value, coordinated services across the healthcare network to effectively manage the health of our community
Expand partnerships	Strengthen relationships with key internal (employees, medical staff) and external (customers, community groups, government organizations, businesses) stakeholders
Grow across the full continuum of care	Build a critical mass of services across the full continuum of care provided by the health system

© 2017 Veralon Partners Inc.

way to the vision, leaving how to achieve them to be determined by the major initiatives and the tactical details in the action plan. An example of the relationship among the three major outputs of strategy formulation—goals, objectives, and major initiatives—from a medical center strategic plan is shown in exhibit 8.10.

Exhibit 8.9: Critical Issues and Key Metrics for Goals: Regional Health System

Critical Issues	Key Metrics for Goals
Coordinate care to deliver value	• Top decile nationally in clinical quality • Top decile nationally in service excellence • Top decile in the state in lowest cost of care • Service area counties perform in the 90th percentile nationally for the majority of health-related indicators
Expand partnerships	• 80% of affiliated providers (e.g., physicians, care extenders) are accountable for performance measures • 25% more incremental providers and staff • "Employer of choice" in the market • 50% increase in annual philanthropic contributions
Grow across the full continuum of care	• Grow net revenue by 25%+ to ensure the appropriate scale to execute strategic initiatives • Increase market share by 5% (on average) across all services • Increase total covered lives by 30%

© 2017 Veralon Partners Inc.

Typically, the result of the task force's strategy formulation process is the identification of 10 to 20 major initiatives for the organization to pursue over the next three to five years in implementing its strategic plan. Because organizations rarely have the resources to pursue so many initiatives vigorously and equally, the strategic planning committee may need to prioritize the initiatives. An example of

Exhibit 8.10: Strategy Recommendations: Our Health System

Goal, 2018	Major Initiatives, 2015–2018
The preferred partner—employee, affiliate, or ally—in the delivery of superior quality and experience for a competitive price	• Transform care and delivery management models (with care partners) • Price competitively • Capture first dollar healthcare spending
Objectives, 2016	• Create an accountable care culture—reward value performance
• Annual associate retention rate improves from 85% to 88% • Covered lives in a risk- or value-based contract increase by 10% • Cost per equivalent discharge is <100% of Medicare	• Integrate functions and key leadership • Manage waste to maximize price leverage

prioritization during a regional referral center's creation of a strategic plan is shown in exhibit 8.11. Such a prioritization process will help set the stage for a realistic and achievable implementation plan. The completion of goals and major initiative setting is significant, in that it puts in place the final piece of the strategic plan with which the board should be principally concerned. Collectively, the mission, vision, strategy, values, goals, and major initiatives constitute the strategic portion of the plan, whereas the remaining components—objectives and actions—are more tactical and operational. It may be helpful to think about the strategic plan as composed of two parts: strategy, which has been the subject of chapters 7 and 8 until this point, and the management action plan, which remains to be completed.

Few not-for-profit boards understand or appreciate the distinction between the strategic and tactical parts of the process. Although

Exhibit 8.11: Example Prioritization of Five-Year Initiatives

Imperative	• Expand primary care network • Continue performance excellence journey • Execute long-range facility plan • Expand workforce development
Critical	• Strengthen clinic relationships • Grow university relationships • Develop centers of excellence • Build ambulatory care clinics • Consider modifying scope of services • Enhance appeal to physicians
Important	• Collaborate with hospital-based physicians • Establish stronger presence in county • Expedite transfers and referrals

Note: Imperative initiatives receive 75% of resources in implementation; critical initiatives receive 20% of resources in implementation (some may need to be deferred); important initiatives receive 5% of resources in implementation (very modest effort or deferral required).

© 2017 Veralon Partners Inc.

the work of the strategic planning committee as a whole should be wrapped up at this point and management should take responsibility for completing the remaining plan tasks and components, most strategic planning committees continue to function in an increasingly dysfunctional way until the plan is complete.

In this situation, a compromise may be in order. Rather than finish the committee's work at this point or allow the committee to continue to provide similar oversight as in prior tasks, the senior management team should thank the committee for completing the overwhelming majority of its important work and offer to reconvene it when the objectives and actions are drafted. Management can then present its draft management action plan and an executive summary of the plan to the committee. Following the committee's review, the action plan and executive summary are submitted to the full board for approval and adoption.

ESTABLISHING OBJECTIVES

If the suggested approach is followed, the remaining planning tasks are carried out under the direction of senior management. These tasks typically involve broader representation of management team members than has been the case up to this point.

Essentially, each goal needs to be dissected into smaller, more manageable components:

- Objectives: short-term targets in each goal area
- Actions: the principal tactics that need to be accomplished to achieve the objectives (and relate to parts of the major initiatives)

The objectives and actions (the latter discussed in chapter 9) collectively compose the near-term game plan to move the organization's strategic plan forward.

Sometimes the objectives are well developed in the critical-issue strategic options and recommendations and task force discussions. In other cases, senior management staff need to determine the objectives, individually or collectively. In either event, the objectives need to provide intermediate, preferably measurable targets on the path to achieving the goals. Review the example of goals and related objectives of one organization shown earlier in exhibit 8.10.

CONTINGENCY PLANNING

Stepping back once or twice during the strategic planning process to consider how the expected direction and strategy will hold up under the likely alternative future conditions identified at the end of the environmental assessment is helpful. Some contingent events may be incorporated explicitly in the strategy formulation process for specific goals and objectives resulting from the barriers and constraints analysis mentioned in exhibit 8.6. Other changes could affect a broad range of strategy formulation outcomes.

Typical contingencies to consider today include the following:

- Shifting national and state policy priorities
- Expedited transition from fee-for-service to value- or risk-based reimbursement, or a reversal of that trend
- Market consolidation, including hospitals, health systems, insurance companies, and physician groups

An example of contingency planning and its impact on the full range of preliminarily defined goals and objectives is illustrated in exhibit 8.12. The example shows how one organization planned for the uncertainty related to healthcare reform in 2008. As a result, the senior management team and the board felt that all reasonable scenarios had been considered and plan implementation moved forward expeditiously and with their full confidence, but with greater ability to adapt should conditions change during implementation. This retrospective examination exemplifies the relationship between the prognostication and the reality that ultimately unfolded. In this case, the forecast description proved to be accurate and thus allowed the system to properly position itself for the future.

FINANCIAL ANALYSIS

One final topic in strategy formulation deserves discussion. A long-standing controversy exists among strategic planners and other healthcare executives about the appropriate depth and breadth of financial analysis in the strategic planning process. William Bellenfant and Matt J. Nelson (2002) suggest that the financial analysis in strategic planning should be "a reality check, ensuring that an organization's strategies do not outstrip its resources and that new initiatives provide the desired level of value." This book recommends a minimalist approach; however, other texts promote the belief that something close to a financial feasibility forecast is necessary.

Exhibit 8.12: Contingency Planning: National Health Reform (from mid-2008 Strategic Plan)

Description	Likelihood	Warning Signs	Implications for System	Readiness/Actions
• Model depends on both political and economic factors • Anticipate phased approach, beginning with extension of coverage to the uninsured with low to medium incomes • May include multistate demonstration projects • Increased regulation to discourage unnecessary use and incentives to address obvious problems such as chronic care • Emphasis on consumer-directed healthcare (HSAs)	• Low to moderate in next five years	• A Democratic president and Democratic majorities in both houses of Congress • Continued pressure to make health insurance affordable even in a resurgent economy • Severe economic distress that increases the number of uninsured • Significant cuts in provider revenue that cause some hospitals to fail and increase pressure for a government bailout • Continuation of dramatic decline in employer-sponsored coverage	• Will force movement from high-margin areas to underserved areas • Greater financial risk to small system hospitals with the exception of some safety net services • Patient safety and outcome criteria will affect both volume and reimbursement	• Improve readiness by building up outpatient business, though this will not optimize revenue in the near term • Ensure systems are in place for managing care, reducing costs of poor quality, reducing variation, and identifying and implementing best practices • Develop a more comprehensive system that improves efficiency and reduces costs • Evaluate current and future impact of HSAs on service lines

Source: Memorial Health System (2008). Used with permission.

Appendix 8.2 offers an example of the recommended level of financial analysis required in a typical strategic planning process.

The strategic plan should have a high-level strategy focus; any substantial financial analysis should occur in implementation or later. However, one note of caution is important. The approach recommended in this book is one that is continually vigilant in recognizing resource limitations, making choices, and focusing effort. This approach can be accomplished with a process that has financial awareness and concerns as parts of its infrastructure so that financial implications are implicitly part of each step of the process. If such high awareness and astuteness is not routinely part of the organization's work, some substantive financial tasks may need to be included in the strategic planning process.

CONCLUSION

When phase 3 is complete, the organization will have a sound framework, through its goals, major initiatives, and objectives, for the work that lies ahead in implementing the plan. But, even more important, if the planning process has been successfully carried out, one of its by-products will be shared learning among organizational leaders about how to address each critical issue. Consensus or near consensus on managing these issues will facilitate problem-free approval of the strategic plan and a rapid transition from planning to implementation.

REFERENCES

Bellenfant, W. L., and M. J. Nelson. 2002. "Strategic Planning: Looking Beyond the Next Move." *hfm*, October, 62–68.
Memorial Health System. 2008. Correspondence with author.
Stony Brook Medicine. 2016. Correspondence with author.
St. Mary's Health. 2015. Correspondence with author.

Example: Issue Documentation

Grove Medical Center (GMC), a midsize community hospital located in the Midwest, identified "physician alignment" as a critical planning issue. A task force charged with developing strategic options and recommendations produced this report for the planning committee.

ISSUE DEFINITION AND SITUATION DESCRIPTION

GMC's medical staff has grown in recent years and now includes a variety of specialties and primary care. While some medical staff members are employed by GMC through Grove Physician Group (GPG), the majority of medical staff members are independent (i.e., in private practice). As the financial environment becomes increasingly challenging, many physicians in GMC's market are seeking closer alignment with hospitals or health systems. The following list includes the factors influencing the market:

- GPG is growing, but there is a need to improve cohesiveness and standardize both clinical and operational processes.
- GMC has limited alternatives for alignment with independent physicians.
- A shortage of primary care physicians in the market exists, and GMC has gaps in several specialty physician services.

- There are some independent physicians in the market that are seeking to align with a health system in some form, but also maintain their private practice.
- Mountainview Health System (MHS), GMC's competition, has been aggressive in acquiring physician practices and is offering participation in its newly developed clinically integrated network.

STRATEGIES EMPLOYED BY OTHERS

Many hospitals across the country are challenged by medical staff alignment issues, including a lack of critical mass in certain specialties, clinical quality or customer service inconsistencies, insufficient care coordination, and frustration in independent practices. These issues commonly linger in an organization because the solutions are perceived to be cost prohibitive. Successful hospitals and health systems use multiple strategies to address alignment concerns, including the following:

- Offer a variety of alignment options, ranging from tighter alignment (e.g., employment, accountable care organization, or clinically integrated network membership) to looser alignment (professional services agreement, information system linkage)
- Provide leadership and professional development opportunities for medical staff members
- Pursue clinical integration, which is a requirement for joint contracting (an increasingly important benefit for physicians)
- Offer incentive-based compensation structures
- Standardize clinical practice procedures and processes and hold medical staff members accountable for quality and patient satisfaction performance

OPTIONS AVAILABLE TO GROVE MEDICAL CENTER

The planning committee considered the options available to GMC. Based on the rapidly evolving market dynamics and the need to respond to physicians' preferences, the members decided that a purposeful and aggressive physician alignment strategy is required for not only continued success, but for ongoing sustainability.

Options	Pros	Cons
1. Pursue an aggressive employment strategy to expand GPG	Tightest form of alignment; counteracts MHS strategy	High cost; significant infrastructure requirements
2. Create a "menu" of alignment options	Appeals to nearly all physicians in the market	Many menu options fall short of meaningful alignment
3. Form a clinically integrated network	Provides financial incentive for alignment without employment hurdles	Time and resource intensive; requires expertise to implement

GMC'S PROPOSED STRATEGY

The proposed strategy calls for GMC to use aspects of options 1 and 2 for a focused employment strategy for specialties that are a high priority for the organization and to offer alternative alignment models targeted to primary care practices. As GMC's number of aligned medical staff members increases, the quality of services provided needs to be standardized while the organization prepares to engage in value-based contract arrangements. The task force developed and presented to the planning committee the following recommendations, goals, objectives, measurement criteria, and barriers.

Recommendation

- Target high-priority specialties for employment in GPG
- Develop several (two or three) alignment alternatives focused on attracting primary care physicians
- Increase physician outreach activity
- Establish clinical and service quality standards, and link physician compensation to performance in these areas

Goals (2016–2020)

- Increase the number of medical staff members in formal economic or clinical alignment relationships by 75 percent
- Coordinate high-quality services across all specialties

Objectives (2016–2017)

- Expand GPG's infrastructure to accommodate planned future growth
- Establish clinical quality and service standards through a collaborative process between administrative and medical staff leaders
- Determine and implement alternative alignment models
- Identify target physician practices for alignment via strategic and financial criteria; align high-priority practices or engage them in discussions with GMC

Measurement Criteria

- Number of physicians in formal alignment arrangements
- GPG revenue

- Clinical quality and service indicators
- Physician engagement survey scores

GMC's Barriers and Constraints

- Resource requirements to acquire high-priority practices
- MHS's aggressive physician employment strategy
- Ability to execute new and unfamiliar alignment models

Example: Strategic Plan Financial Analysis

At the outset of its strategic planning process, GMC recognized that its baseline operating income estimates (exhibit A.1) would not allow it to achieve its vision. After identifying initiatives in phase 3 of its strategic planning process, GMC estimated the financial impact of each (exhibit A.2) and determined that the initiatives were not expected to generate the required financial improvement. Several initiatives were then reconsidered and refined to achieve the desired financial result.

Exhibit A.1: Strategic Financial Analysis Projected Baseline Income Statement

	Budgeted Fiscal Year 2016	Projected Fiscal Year 2020
Revenue	$492,230	$599,460
Expenses	$495,840	$601,260
Operating income	($3,610)	($1,800)
Operating margin	(0.73%)	(0.30%)
Non–operating gains	$4,930	$5,410
Net income	$1,320	$3,610
Net margin	0.27%	0.60%

Note: Dollars in thousands.

Exhibit A.2: Net Financial Impact from Major Initiatives

	Fiscal Year 2016	Fiscal Year 2017	Fiscal Year 2018	Fiscal Year 2019	Fiscal Year 2020	Net Impact from Major Initiatives
Baseline net income	$1.3	$1.5	$2.1	$2.8	$3.6	
Estimated impact from major initiatives						
IP volume growth	$0.1	$0.3	$0.6	$1.0	$1.5	$3.5
Ambulatory surgery volume growth	$0.2	$0.3	$0.5	$0.7	$1.0	$2.7
Downstream ancillary volume growth	$0.5	$0.9	$1.4	$1.8	$2.0	$6.0
Technology investments	($0.5)	($0.5)	($0.5)	($0.5)	($0.5)	($2.5)
Other infrastructure investment	($0.8)	($0.8)	($0.8)	($0.8)	($0.8)	($4.0)
Revised net income	$0.8	$1.7	$3.3	$5.0	$6.8	$5.7

Note: Dollars in millions.

© 2017 Veralon Partners Inc.

CHAPTER 9

Phase 4: Transition to Implementation

When it comes to getting things done, we need fewer architects and more bricklayers.

—*Colleen C. Barrett (attributed)*

Never confuse movement with action.

—*Ernest Hemingway*

No strategic planning topic today is more controversial than how to manage successfully the transition from planning to implementation. While developing a good strategic plan is difficult, many feel that implementation is by far more challenging. The transition from strategic planning to implementation is a point at which plans frequently stray off course.

A study of healthcare strategic planning in 2005–2006 revealed that while the core strategic plan development tasks were perceived by senior leaders as being carried out well or very well, implementation planning, implementation itself, and communication of the strategic plan inside and outside of the organization were cited as areas in which significant improvement could and should occur (Zuckerman 2007).

Most experts concur with Peter M. Ginter, W. Jack Duncan, and Linda E. Swayne (2013, 400), who postulate that "effective strategy implementation requires the same determination and effort that is devoted to situation analysis and strategy formulation."

More specifically, Martin Corboy and Diarmaid O Corrbui (1999, 29–30) identify the following "seven deadly sins . . . that doom effective strategy implementation":

1. *The strategy is lacking in terms of rigor, insight, vision, ambition, or practicality.* If the strategy is simply more of the same, comfortable, and incremental, it will not create the excitement needed for successful implementation.

2. *People are not sure how the strategy is to be implemented.* Leaders are too impatient to make the strategy happen, so they don't communicate details about how implementation is to proceed. They sometimes consider communication to be time-consuming indecisiveness.

3. *The strategy is communicated on a need-to-know basis.* It is not disseminated freely throughout the organization.

4. *Some or all aspects of strategy implementation lack a specific person in charge.* Failure to carefully manage all aspects of implementation results in oversights and confusion.

5. *Strategic leaders send mixed signals by dropping out of sight when implementation begins.* The absence of strategic leadership implies that implementation is not worthy of leaders' attention and, therefore, unimportant.

6. *Unforeseen obstacles to implementation occur.* When they do, responsible people are not prepared to overcome them in creative and innovative ways.

7. *Strategy becomes all-consuming,* and details of day-to-day operations are lost or neglected. Strategy is important, but so are operations.

The focus of this chapter is to provide guidance for transitioning effectively from planning to implementation. Exhibit 9.1 highlights several key elements of this final activity of the strategic planning process: the importance of increased involvement of those who

Exhibit 9.1: Developing the Plan: Action Planning

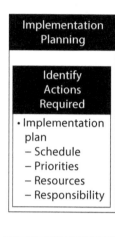

Implementation Planning

Identify Actions Required

• Implementation plan
 – Schedule
 – Priorities
 – Resources
 – Responsibility

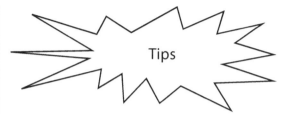

Tips

• Increased involvement of clinicians and managers in this activity, which makes it highly desirable
• Before completion of the plan, an ongoing progress tracking system should be defined and agreed on by leadership
• Corporate sets priorities, especially among competing resource needs of operating units

will be important participants in implementation of the plan, the need to specify and adhere to an ongoing tracking system for plan implementation, and the critical role in larger healthcare systems of the corporate organization in defining and mediating demands for resources required to carry out implementation.

The five major activities involved in a successful transition from planning to implementation are briefly described in the following section, succeeded by a more detailed discussion of each in subsequent sections of this chapter.

DEVELOP A DETAILED YEAR 1 IMPLEMENTATION PLAN FOR THE NEW STRATEGIC PLAN

Strategic goals, objectives, and major initiatives developed during strategy formulation must be operationalized through a set of tactics with associated time frames and standards of accountability that serve as the implementation road map and link with budget-development activities for year 1.

- *Prepare and submit the proposed strategic plan to the board of directors for review and approval.* Depending on the full board's level of participation in the strategic plan development process, one to three working sessions to present key findings, discuss future market assumptions, and review proposed strategic priorities might be required prior to board adoption.
- *Roll out the new strategic plan to internal and external audiences.* Organizational leaders should prepare a comprehensive communication plan that is ready to go once board approval has been obtained, including the identification of target audiences, key messages, and presentation materials.
- *Establish systems for monitoring and reporting progress.* Tracking changes in key metrics via a formal reporting system and timetable helps to maintain the focus on strategic priorities, instill accountability for results, and prompt midcourse corrections to get back on track as conditions warrant.
- *Update the strategic plan on a regular basis, no less than annually.* In today's dynamic world of healthcare, organizational strategy must be flexible enough to accommodate unanticipated changes in the environment—unforeseen challenges as well as opportunities. Strategic priorities should be revisited at least annually, so that important adjustments can be made when necessary.

The development of a detailed first-year implementation plan is a critical component of transitioning successfully from planning to action. This task involves translating the strategic goals, objectives, and major initiatives developed during strategy formulation (see chapter 8) into a set of thoughtful activities that will lead to progress toward a set of desired outcomes. Exhibit 9.2 illustrates the cascading

Exhibit 9.2: Relationship Between Strategy and Implementation

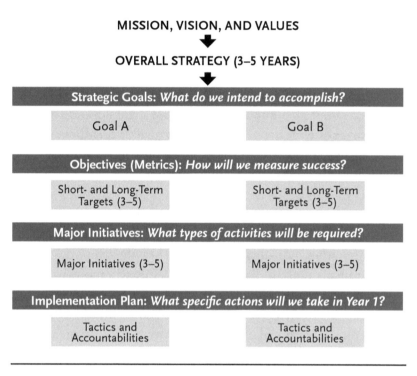

MISSION, VISION, AND VALUES
⬇

OVERALL STRATEGY (3–5 YEARS)
⬇

Strategic Goals: *What do we intend to accomplish?*

| Goal A | Goal B |

Objectives (Metrics): *How will we measure success?*

| Short- and Long-Term Targets (3–5) | Short- and Long-Term Targets (3–5) |

Major Initiatives: *What types of activities will be required?*

| Major Initiatives (3–5) | Major Initiatives (3–5) |

Implementation Plan: *What specific actions will we take in Year 1?*

| Tactics and Accountabilities | Tactics and Accountabilities |

© 2017 Veralon Partners Inc.

relationship between the strategy formulation outputs and the year 1 implementation plan.

During the course of the strategic plan development process, primary responsibility shifts from the board, whose focus is on overall strategic direction ("Where do we need to go?"), to the senior management team, whose responsibility is to make it happen ("How will we get there?"). Development of the initial-year and subsequent-year implementation plans, therefore, rests with the senior management team.

Exhibit 9.3 provides an example of content for a specific strategic goal, including short- and long-term objectives, major initiatives, and year 1 implementation activities and accountabilities. In this section, we suggest that senior management use a four-step process to create a compelling and effective implementation plan.

- Step 1: For each strategic goal, appoint one or more executive champions from the senior management team to draft the year 1 implementation plan. The executive champions then assemble a team of individuals to assist with the process for each goal. Depending on the complexity of the assigned area and scope of implementation activities required, the team may consist of as few as 2 to 3 individuals or as many as 20. At this point, it is appropriate and advisable to broaden team membership to include middle managers and other individuals likely to be heavily involved in implementation. Each team ordinarily will meet two or three times to flesh out the initial implementation details for its assigned goal. The example shown in exhibit 9.3 contains minimal details, which will be fine for many organizations, but others may prefer to break down tactics into smaller steps and time frames.
- Step 2: Each team reviews its respective draft goal statement, objectives, and major initiatives for clarity, alignment, and completeness. As shown in exhibit 9.3, each team should begin by carefully reviewing, and refining as necessary, the proposed framework developed thus far to make sure it is clear and compelling. Does the goal statement clearly explain what the organization wants to achieve? Have short-term and long-term objectives been identified, and are they quantifiable? Do the major initiatives lend themselves to specific activities that will move the needle on achieving the proposed goal and objectives? Note that the component most often needing additional work by the team is defining and quantifying the objectives. What exactly will you measure, and what

will be the source for the data? Do you have baseline data to know where you are starting from? What should the future targets be and why? It is important that the teams refrain from jumping to step 3 until step 2 has been completed.

- Step 3: Each team identifies a set of proposed projects and tactics to be undertaken during year 1 of implementation. The group needs to delineate specific tactics the organization will engage in during the year, as well as the expected time frame for each tactic (Will it be completed in the 12-month period?), the individual with lead responsibility, and a high-level estimate of resource requirements and expected impact. It is better (and usually more challenging) to identify a limited number of tactics that collectively will result in significant impact, rather than a long list of projects that provide limited return on investment.

- Step 4: Senior management reviews all draft implementation plans to ensure internal alignment with appropriate prioritization and allocation of resources. After all teams have completed their proposed year 1 implementation plans, senior management is responsible for evaluating the plan in its entirety. Are any of the proposed tactics in conflict with other tactics? Are there areas of overlapping tactics that need to be clarified? Does the organization have the resources to take on all suggested tactics in year 1, or should some be deferred for a later time? Most important, if all items identified in the implementation plan are accomplished, does it significantly advance the organization toward its strategic goals and objectives?

A couple of additional thoughts are in order at this point about the importance of creating buy-in for implementation. The initial framework of the strategic plan (goals, objectives, major initiatives)

Exhibit 9.3: Strategic Goal with Detailed Objectives and Year 1 Implementation Plan

Strategic Goal #1

Our health system successfully participates in alternative reimbursement models that emphasize coordinated and longitudinal care for patients

Objectives for Strategic Goal #1

	1-Year Target	5-Year Target
Reduction in inpatient stays for ambulatory sensitive conditions	–10%	–30%
Reduction in readmission rates	–10%	–40%
Reduction in per member cost of care for ACO attributed lives	–5%	–15%
Positive overall operating margin from risk-based reimbursement contracts	2%	5%
Growth in total net revenue attributed to risk-based reimbursement models	+10%	+60%

Major Initiatives for Strategic Goal #1

- Refine care models to focus on providing "Right care, Right time, Right place"
- Improve coordination and efficacy across care locations—within our system and with external partners
- Enhance operational capabilities to assume financial risk under alternative reimbursement models
- Seek out new and expanded opportunities to participate in alternative reimbursement models

(continued)

Implementation Plan for Year 1

Projects and Tactics for Year 1	Time Frame	Lead	Resource Requirements[1]	Estimated Impact[2]
Implement three new care coordinator positions for primary care offices	Q1	JS	Medium	High
Implement nurse hotline service for ACO members	Q2	JS	Low	Medium
Utilize ACO data to identify opportunities to improve care delivery	Q1–Q4	GJ	Low	Medium
Institute Lean as a means for streamlining and improving care processes	Q1–Q4	SD	Medium	Medium
Improve continuity of patient care by providing community partners with an appropriate level of access to patient information	Q3	GJ	Low	Medium
Develop cost accounting system	Q3–Q4	BL	High	Medium
Pursue bundled payments for selected procedures	Q3–Q4	DD	Medium	Low
Explore opportunities for alternative reimbursement contracts with commercial payers	Q3–Q4	DD	Low	Low

[1]Time and/or financial resources: Low=0.50 person days and/or <$250K during the year; Medium=50–100 person days and/or $250K–$500K; High=100+ person days and/or >$500K

[2]Net impact from incremental revenue and/or decreased costs: Low=<$100K during the year; Medium=$100K–$500K, High=>$500K

© 2017 Veralon Partners Inc.

is developed largely by the board and senior management, but one key to successful implementation is commitment at the operations level, primarily with middle management. To facilitate buy-in and make sure implementation expectations are realistic, those managers need to actively participate in shaping the parts of the plan for which they will be principally responsible (i.e., actions, schedule).

Another important recommendation is to proceed with actual implementation as quickly as possible to avoid losing momentum. Multiple tactics and projects can typically be initiated even before the strategic plan is formally adopted by the board, with adjustments made down the road, as necessary, to maintain consistency with the final version of the plan.

BOARD REVIEW AND APPROVAL OF THE STRATEGIC PLAN

Following completion of the year 1 implementation plan, submit the new strategic plan to the board of directors for review, discussion, and consideration for approval. If planning activities have proceeded smoothly up until this point, adoption of the strategic plan is fairly straightforward. In this section, we discuss five recommended steps in the board review and approval process.

Step 1: Prepare the Draft Strategic Plan Document and Presentation Materials

Preparing two versions of the strategic plan is helpful—a three- to five-page executive summary that can be used as a stand-alone document, as well as a more comprehensive version that contains more extensive documentation.

In the rush to move from planning to implementation, organizations sometimes overlook the need for an executive summary. However, this document is often the only strategic plan output read by board members and other important stakeholders. When new board members and senior executives join the organization, the executive summary of the strategic plan provides an insightful snapshot of current challenges and strategic priorities. The executive summary should include the rationale for preparation of the strategic plan, an overview of the planning process, key findings, and a summary of proposed strategic goals, objectives, and major initiatives. Exhibits 9.4 and 9.5 present samples of summary strategic plan documents. Some organizations issue the executive summary as a discrete document, while others place it as the first section in the complete strategic plan report. Appendix 9.1 represents an example of a more comprehensive strategic plan document.

In addition to the executive summary, organizational leaders should prepare a full strategic plan report at the conclusion of the planning process. This document should include the output of all planning activities and a description of important process steps (e.g., interviews, retreats). This document serves as the record for all that occurred during the planning process and as a reference source for analyses and supporting information that may be germane to implementation.

Step 2: Obtain a Resolution by the Strategic Planning Committee Recommending Board Approval of the Plan

Although it may only be a formality if the strategic planning process has proceeded smoothly, nearly all healthcare organizations convene the strategic planning committee for a final meeting to review the draft plan and recommend adoption to the board. After making any additional refinements in wording or format, the committee passes a resolution to forward the draft strategic plan to the board for review and consideration for approval. The final meeting can also be used to discuss next steps and implementation and to outline how the

Exhibit 9.4: Sample Summary of Overall Strategic Direction for McDonough District Hospital (MDH)

Organizational Direction

DESIRED FUTURE STATE

— Key stakeholders (board members, physicians, employees) aligned and committed to a *shared vision*

— *Strong primary care base* aligned with MDH and integrated in the community

— *Specialty physician services* that provide value and are *sustainable*

— *Inpatient volume and market share* stabilized and *trending upward*

— *Operating independently* with a *strong financial position*

— *Multiple partnerships/collaborations* to ensure that community needs are met and MDH is viewed as a strong community partner

MISSION STATEMENT

The mission of McDonough District Hospital, in partnership with its Medical Staff, is to provide health services with a personal approach to care that enhances the quality of life.

VISION STATEMENT

To be your First Choice for First Class Health Services.

VALUES

HONESTY AND INTEGRITY – RESPECT – EXCEPTIONAL SERVICE – COMMITMENT TO EXCELLENCE AND TEAMWORK

(continued)

(continued from previous page)

3-Year Strategic Goals and Major Initiatives

GOALS	MAJOR INITIATIVES
1 **FOUNDATIONAL STRATEGIES** Maintain excellence in hospital operations, infrastructure, and financial performance as foundational strategies for future growth and development	• Ensure the availability of a high-quality workforce and medical staff • Achieve ongoing improvements in quality, patient safety, and patient satisfaction • Maintain a strong financial position • Provide up-to-date facilities and technology • Forge strong connections with the communities we serve
2 **SCALE AND SCOPE** Achieve thoughtful and sustainable growth in scale and scope of services	• Increase the availability of both primary care and physician specialty services based on community need and operational viability • Expand outpatient services when appropriate and feasible—new and wider distribution of services • Reduce patient outmigration for inpatient care that we can provide locally • Work with partners to address gaps in non–acute care services; prevention/wellness through post-acute care
3 **PATIENT AND CONSUMER FOCUS** Redesign care delivery models to meet the changing expectations of our patients and communities	• Improve access to timely and convenient care • Increase transparency in pricing, quality, and patient safety • Facilitate multiple ways for patients to provide input about their satisfaction with and expectations for care delivery • Engage patients and families as partners in their healthcare
4 **SHARED VISION AND TEAMWORK** Create a shared vision for MDH that resonates throughout the organization, inspires teamwork, and promotes professional camaraderie	• Generate support for a unified vision that positions MDH for continued long-term success • Invest in leadership development for management and medical staff • Strengthen employee and physician engagement with MDH • Align internal policies and processes to support organizational values and priorities
5 **POPULATION HEALTH** Position MDH to be successful in the transition to alternative payment models based on coordinated and longitudinal care	• Refine care models to focus on providing "Right care, Right time, Right place" • Improve coordination and efficiency across care locations—with MDH and with external partners • Pursue opportunities to participate in alternative payment models as appropriate

committee will be involved in subsequent strategic plan updates or implementation monitoring.

Step 3: Provide an Opportunity for Medical Staff Review and Input (for Hospitals and Health Systems)

Prior to final approval, most hospital and health system boards want to see some level of medical staff review and feedback on the draft strategic plan as a part of the process, although there is substantial variation in how organizations approach that task.

Medical staff participation in this stage may range from a few individual or small-group meetings with physician leaders (especially in highly competitive environments) to meetings with the medical executive committee or other medical leadership groups to broad-based input with widespread participation. The purpose of the dialogue with the medical staff is to obtain high-level feedback as opposed to a more detailed or parochial discussion, although some of that will likely occur anyway. Finally, unless the board directs otherwise, it is important to communicate that the requested role of the medical staff is to offer perspectives on the draft strategic plan, rather than approval.

Step 4: Hold Formal and Informal Work Sessions with the Board to Review and Discuss the Proposed Strategic Plan

In most healthcare organizations, at least one presentation of the complete draft strategic plan to the board is scheduled prior to formal review and consideration for approval. This educational session, which is frequently conducted in a retreat setting, provides an opportunity for the full board to review and question the plan's analyses, findings, and recommendations. The purpose is to increase the board's understanding of the plan and its implications for the organization, and to allow any important issues about the development process and subsequent implementation to surface and be resolved.

For most organizations, this one educational session is the only major activity required before the board feels prepared to formally consider the proposed plan for approval. At times, however, the board may require additional time and discussion to become comfortable with the plan before taking formal action. In that case, it is usually productive to schedule another educational session, small group discussions, or one-on-one meetings between board members and the CEO before proceeding further. Senior management and leaders of the strategic planning committee need to do whatever is necessary to ensure that board members understand and support the strategic plan. They should be especially sensitive to board members' concerns, confusion, or discomfort and attempt to address each board member's needs, so that the full board is genuinely enthusiastic about strategic plan adoption and implementation.

Step 5: Board Votes to Adopt the Strategic Plan

The board's review and approval process of the strategic plan may encompass a limited number of steps carried out over a few weeks, or a significant number of steps over a few months. This variation is largely a function of the complexity of the plan, its recommendations, and organizational style, such as the degree of deliberateness in the review and approval process.

Rarely are strategic plans not approved, although there are instances where the plan is rejected by the board or returned to the planning staff or committee for major reworking. When the staff, senior management, and strategic planning committee have done their jobs well, including gathering extensive input and communicating effectively throughout the plan development process,

Exhibit 9.5: Strategic Plan Summary

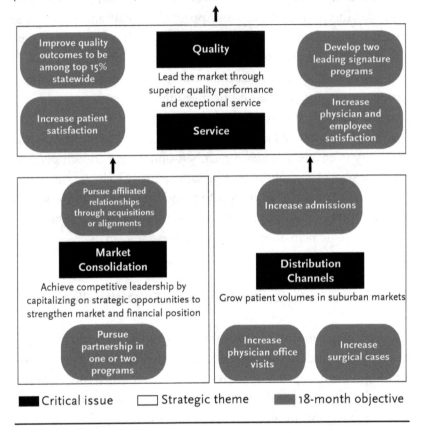

OHS Organizational Direction

Our Health System will be the healthcare leader in the region, providing exceptional medical care and service for every patient, every day, in a patient-centered, family-focused environment.

Quality

Lead the market through superior quality performance and exceptional service

Service

Improve quality outcomes to be among top 15% statewide

Increase patient satisfaction

Develop two leading signature programs

Increase physician and employee satisfaction

Pursue affiliated relationships through acquisitions or alignments

Market Consolidation

Achieve competitive leadership by capitalizing on strategic opportunities to strengthen market and financial position

Pursue partnership in one or two programs

Increase admissions

Distribution Channels

Grow patient volumes in suburban markets

Increase physician office visits

Increase surgical cases

■ Critical issue ☐ Strategic theme ■ 18-month objective

board approval should proceed without any serious roadblocks. If the strategic plan is not adopted when brought forward for formal consideration, it is likely that either appropriate preparation did not occur or sensitivity to board concerns was lacking.

STRATEGIC PLAN ROLLOUT AND COMMUNICATION

The next key element of a successful transition from strategic planning to implementation is a strong communications process. Some organizations do an exceptionally good job of communicating the results of strategic planning and moving into the implementation phase, while others do not.

Few would argue against the importance of communicating the results of strategic planning as a critical component of the transition from planning to implementation—so why is there such wide variation in attention to this task? What appears to be at issue is the degree of formality and the extent of the communications process, as well as the rigor and need for structure in transitioning to implementation.

Organizations that move smoothly and effectively from planning to implementation communicate broadly and use completion of the strategic plan to signal to key stakeholders that a new era is beginning. The use of celebration as a communications element garners attention and interest and raises expectations.

The communications process should inform and involve constituents. By sharing strategic plan findings, recommendations, implementation priorities, and sequencing of major initiatives with key individuals and groups, the prospects for plan acceptance and implementation support are enhanced.

C. Davis Fogg (2010) outlines some of the most important considerations in designing and effectively carrying out a strategic plan communications process. The following section discusses three central aspects of the communications plan.

1. Audiences that need to be addressed
   - Senior management and boards
   - Their subordinates

- Other employees (in most healthcare organizations, medical staff members and key external constituencies)
2. How to frame the message for each audience
   - Tailor information to their jobs and positions.
   - Take into account the information that they need to carry out their part in the plan.
   - Be sensitive to their need to know proprietary information or planned strategies.

   As a general rule, the more people know about the vision and strategic plan, their role in it, and its effect on their job, the better. This knowledge helps direct spontaneous action, plans, and programs at lower levels in the organization. It also reduces working at cross-purposes and misunderstandings about what is strategically important (e.g., quality vs. cost reductions).
3. The best method of communicating the plan
   - Develop scripts and visual aids for each major target audience so that a uniform message is conveyed.
   - Have a senior manager, preferably a member of the planning team, present the plan to each target group.
   - Leave time for employees (and others) to ask questions and get answers, preferably in small groups facilitated by managers who are also recording issues.

Refer to the ideas listed in exhibit 9.6 as potential strategies and materials to incorporate into a comprehensive communications plan. Appendix 9.1 provides an example of a strategic plan summary document that was developed by an organization as a communications tool to share with key constituencies. When developing written materials about an organization's strategic priorities and plans, senior leaders must balance the desire and need to share enough information to create buy-in and enthusiasm with the risk of compromising competitive advantage by prematurely divulging too much information.

Exhibit 9.6: Potential Ideas to Incorporate into Communications Plan

Internal Communications	External Communications
• Communicate directly with frontline employees as often as possible to ensure buy-in of strategic initiatives • Train executives and managers to convey strategic initiatives and core values in a consistent manner • Articulate accountability so that staff members have a clear understanding of responsibilities • Reinforce strategic initiatives through symbolic representation, such as posters or signs • Use multiple networks: town hall meetings, employee newsletters, intranet postings, webcasts/podcasts • Consider producing a video with staff at all levels explaining the plan	• Create summary document for marketing materials and media distribution • Post succinct and clear outline of strategic plan on website • Create presentation with a review of strategic plan for CEO to give to community groups • Schedule appearances before various community constituencies (e.g., church groups, chamber of commerce)

A well-organized communications plan will be an essential part of the strategic plan rollout.

© 2017 Veralon Partners Inc.

Fogg (2010) also suggests that strategic plan communication is not a one-time event and that consistent effort and attention of the CEO and senior management are necessary to carrying out this task successfully. While the planning process may be technically complete when the board approves the strategic plan, all of the hard and creative work may be for naught if these efforts are not complemented by a solid communications plan.

SYSTEMS FOR MONITORING AND REPORTING PROGRESS

Every organization should develop a formal system for monitoring and reporting progress even before the strategic plan is approved. In the first year of implementation, many organizations monitor progress on a monthly or every-other-month basis. Assuming good progress is being made and significant external or internal changes are not occurring, formal progress tracking and monitoring may be conducted with decreasing frequency, but it probably needs to occur at least quarterly if it is to remain effective. Please refer to the next chapter for a detailed discussion and specific format suggestions regarding progress reports. Tracking and reporting progress are related to reviewing and updating the plan, both of which are discussed in the next chapter.

CONCLUSION

This chapter addresses a successful transition from planning to implementation and completion of the strategic plan. A thorough, structured approach to this transition is recommended in five key steps:

1. Develop a detailed year 1 implementation plan for the new strategic plan.
2. Prepare and submit the proposed strategic plan to the board of directors for review and approval.
3. Roll out the new strategic plan to internal and external audiences.

4. Establish systems for monitoring and reporting progress.
5. Update the strategic plan on a regular basis, no less than annually.

Because the transition from planning to implementation is especially difficult for many healthcare organizations, a leadership-driven, carefully managed, and clearly articulated approach to this phase is required. As a result, the transition should be smoother, and it should position the organization for a higher degree of implementation success.

REFERENCES

Corboy, M., and D. O Corrbui. 1999. "The Seven Deadly Sins of Strategy." *Management Accounting* 77 (10): 29–33.

Fogg, C. D. 2010. *Team-Based Strategic Planning: A Complete Guide to Structuring, Facilitating, and Implementing the Process.* N. p.: CreateSpace Independent Publishing Platform.

Ginter, P. M., W. J. Duncan, and L. E. Swayne. 2013. *Strategic Management of Health Care Organizations*, 7th ed. San Francisco: Jossey-Bass.

Zuckerman, A. M. 2007. *Raising the Bar: Best Practices for Healthcare Strategic Planning.* Chicago: Society for Healthcare Strategy & Market Development, American Hospital Association.

Regional Health System

2017-2022 Strategic Plan

Regional
Health

Regional
Health

INTRODUCTION

- Regional Health is a first generation integrated delivery system. It has annual revenues of about $1.2B and consists of five hospitals, including a large tertiary medical center, an employed medical group with about 300 providers, and an insurance company with 150,000 members.
- Regional Health is based in a small city, but serves a large rural geographic area of about 1,000,000 residents It competes with a not-for-profit community hospital, two smaller for-profit hospitals that are part of national chains, a statewide Blue Cross plan, other national insurance companies and a variety of niche players. Regional's recent expansion initiatives have strained relations with smaller providers and communities in the region.
- With the recent arrival of a new CEO, Regional began a comprehensive strategic planning effort
- Major activities in the strategic planning process included:
  - Conducting 125 stakeholder interviews
  - Evaluating 600 survey responses from three stakeholder groups (management, board, physicians)
  - Assessing each business entity within the Regional Health structure
  - Facilitating input sessions with medical staff leaders and subsidiary boards
  - Holding monthly working sessions with the strategic planning committee

---

Regional
Health

FACTORS DRIVING THE NEED FOR CHANGE, 2017-2022

Consumerism: publicly available information will increasingly influence consumer choice; quality, service, and cost will become more significant considerations for patients when selecting providers

Healthcare Value = $\frac{\text{Quality of Care}}{\text{Cost of Care}}$

Delivering value: reimbursement methodologies will be more significantly tied to outcomes; greater integration of system components will be necessary to provide care efficiently

Reimbursement: modest increases at best; cost-shifting to commercial plans to subsidize low payments from other payers will diminish; continuing pressure to reduce costs

Scale and scope: Regional Health needs to scale up and develop differentiated centers of excellence to compete successfully with national organizations and niche players

These external environmental factors were key drivers in the identification of the areas of focus that Regional Health must address

Regional
Health

ORGANIZATIONAL DIRECTION

OUR MISSION

Regional Health improves the health and well-being of the people and communities we serve

OUR VISION

In partnership with others, Regional Health will lead the way to better health

OUR VALUES

CARING – We are compassionate and caring

INTEGRITY – We treat others with integrity and respect

COLLABORATION – We collaborate with our customers, peers, partners and communities

EXCELLENCE – We strive for excellence in all we do

Overall Strategy: Regional Health will position itself as a market innovator and differentiate from others based on value

---

Regional
Health

THREE BROAD STRATEGIC GOALS FOR THE NEXT FIVE YEARS

Coordinate care to deliver value

DELIVER HIGH-VALUE, COORDINATED SERVICES ACROSS THE HEALTH CARE NETWORK TO EFFECTIVELY MANAGE THE HEALTH OF OUR COMMUNITY

Expand partnerships

STRENGTHEN RELATIONSHIPS WITH KEY INTERNAL (EMPLOYEES, MEDICAL STAFF MEMBERS) AND EXTERNAL STAKEHOLDERS (CUSTOMERS, COMMUNITY GROUPS, GOVERNMENT ORGANIZATIONS AND BUSINESSES)

Grow across the full continuum of care

BUILD A CRITICAL MASS OF SERVICES ACROSS THE FULL CONTINUUM OF CARE

5

Regional Health

SUMMARY OF MAJOR INITIATIVES

FY2017	FY2018	FY2019	FY2020	FY2021	FY2022

Coordinate care to deliver value

- Develop a system-wide framework for managing populations and coordinating care, with a focus on improving operational efficiency, reducing unnecessary care, and using evidence-based protocols
- Strengthen EMR and analytical capabilities to improve care management and outcomes
- Engage medical staff in creating systems of shared accountability for performance indicators – clinical, patient experience and financial
- Provide education for patients and families to take charge of their personal health
- Continue to develop population health capabilities, including arrangements that involve shared financial risk

Expand partnerships

- Develop an array of options for physician alignment
- Leverage relationship with academic partner to expand scope of services
- Formalize educational training programs for nursing and allied health personnel
- Update approaches to employee recruitment and retention to better attract top talent
- Implement systematic and proven approaches to philanthropy that for increased donations

Grow across the full continuum of care

- Expand continuum of care services to better meet community needs
- Strengthen regional referrals for tertiary services
- Increase number of insured lives with targeted geographic and product development strategies
- Enhance geographic distribution of ambulatory services
- Create innovations lab for testing new approaches to care delivery

6

Regional Health

METRICS FOR MEASURING PROGRESS

FY2017	FY2018	FY2019	FY2020	FY2021	FY2022

Coordinate care to deliver value

- Top decile nationally in clinical quality
- Top decile nationally in service excellence
- Top decile in the state in lowest cost of care
- Service area counties perform in the 90th percentile nationally for the majority of health-related indicators

Expand partnerships

- 80% of affiliated providers (physicians, care extenders, etc.) are accountable for performance measures
- 25% more incremental providers and staff
- "Employer of choice" in the market
- 50% increase in annual philanthropic contributions

Grow across the full continuum of care

- Grow net revenue by 25%+ to ensure the appropriate scale for executing strategic initiatives
- Increase market share by 5% (on average) across all services
- Increase total covered lives by 30%

7

CHAPTER 10

Annual Review and Update

Even if you're on the right track, you'll get run over if you just sit there.

—*Will Rogers (attributed)*

In today's healthcare delivery environment, a meaningful strategic planning process should result in a plan that has a useful life of at least three years—perhaps five in less competitive markets or those with a slow-to-moderate pace of change. This time line appears to parallel the general business world, wherein it is typical that a comprehensive plan update or overhaul is required about every four to five years (Fogg 2010). Regardless of the specific planning horizon, the plan should be reviewed no less than annually, focusing on whether the intended results are being achieved and to what extent. This step is important—not only to keep abreast of progress and manage performance but also to stay attuned to the environment, to maintain momentum for execution, and because doing so is viewed positively by potential partners, bond rating agencies, regulatory bodies, and other external stakeholders. Some innovations to the review process that may provide a stronger foundation for sustainable execution are described in more detail in chapter 11.

The annual review entails a high-level evaluation of progress toward the vision and goal achievement, and the annual update makes appropriate adjustments to ensure relevance of goals based on the pace and amount of progress made and in light of significant changes in the market, regulations, and the industry, as well as any major internal changes. The outcome of the annual review may be a substantial update to the plan, however. Typically, for at least one and often for two years after a comprehensive strategic planning process has been completed, a far less extensive update is called for. If it is unlikely that a robust update of the plan will be warranted, any refresh is done only to facilitate a productive review process and to inform next year's action plan. This action plan, like the one developed after full plan completion and as described in chapter 9, should identify appropriate projects and tactics for the coming year, project leads, anticipated time frames, required resources, and expected impact.

Organizations should be clear on how much and what type of process is called for and be thorough but judicious in determining the degree of update warranted for each of the four main phases of the plan (the following sections provide guidance on making these decisions). As a general rule of thumb, a routine review and update should require one-quarter of the effort of the initial plan (Fogg 2010).

REVIEW AND UPDATE APPROACH

Preliminary Assessment

To conduct a focused review and update, it is helpful to set the stage by gauging progress to date, degree of change since plan completion, and continued relevance of key plan elements. The following set of questions (and answers) is very useful to preliminarily identify how much of an update is called for and what kind of preparation and process may be most applicable:

- Have we made sufficient progress toward each of our strategic goals in the past year as measured by our performance on year 1 objectives?
- Are there recent or pending developments (internally or externally) that have or will have a *major* impact on organizational direction and priorities?

- Do current goals and metrics still reflect our most important strategic aims?
- Do major initiatives still represent the key ways we will pursue our goals?

Exhibit 10.1 shows select possible scenarios for answering the four questions and provides insight into how answers translate to the degree and type of update required. While not an exhaustive set of scenarios by any means, it is helpful to see that patterns of answers emerge from asking these questions. For example, if insignificant internal and external change has occurred since the development of the last full plan, and even if progress to date on the plan has not been exceptional, an extensive update is unlikely to be required. On the other hand, even if progress on the existing plan has been adequate, a high degree of change may meaningfully reduce the relevancy of goals and major initiatives and thus create the need to update more extensively.

Using the questions and your answers in conjunction with the framework should give you a baseline sense of how much updating will be required, which in turn will inform how much preparation and process is needed.

Organizing and Setting Expectations

No matter how much updating is required, the process and outcomes of both the review and update should be recorded and maintained. Documentation is especially critical if a substantive update is in order, as it will likely be necessary to obtain formal board input on and approval of modifications.

As with the comprehensive planning process, the review and update processes are most efficient and productive when preparation is done in advance. Of the four key categories of preparation outlined in chapter 3—communication and expectations, management and leadership, context, and mind-set—the first three, and only specific steps in each, are most relevant to the review and update processes.

Exhibit 10.1: Preliminary Assessment to Determine Annual Update Approach

	Potential Answer Scenarios			
	Scenario 1	Scenario 2	Scenario 3	Scenario 4
1. Good progress?	Y	N	N	Y or N
2. Lots of change?	N	N	Y	Y
3. Goals still relevant?	Y	Y	Y (Mostly)	N
4. Initiatives still appropriate?	Y	Y	N	N
Updating Required	Minimal	Minimal	Moderate	Significant
Approach	• Informal update process; focus on action plan revisions • Affirm plan conclusions and recommendations • Develop new action plan; make sure next year's objectives are appropriately aggressive based on progress to date	• Informal update process; focus on action plan revisions • Affirm plan conclusions and recommendations • Develop new action plan that is more structured with clearer accountability and more consistent progress checks	• Formal but somewhat abbreviated update process • Update environmental assessment outputs • Tweak goals and metrics; revise major initiatives • Develop new action plan	• Formal and lengthy update process • Update outputs of environmental assessment and strategy formulation, including drafting new major initiatives • Review organizational direction (primarily to affirm but modify as necessary) • Develop new action plan

© 2017 Veralon Partners Inc.

1. *Communication and expectations.* The step of primary importance in this category for the review and update is defining desired outcomes. In cases where minimal updating is anticipated, the annual update should yield changes sufficient to justify continuing per the original plan. Typical desired outcomes in these circumstances include a thorough understanding of progress to date and successful execution of fairly minor course corrections. When significant change has occurred, plan implementation never started in earnest or has stalled, or the organization is in crisis, the annual update must be designed to yield more effective outcomes that restore plan relevancy, reset priorities, and incite more or different action.

2. *Management and leadership.* The key to this category is defining roles and responsibilities of the leadership and management team. The extent to which executive leadership and the board are actively involved should correlate to the degree of update deemed necessary. If the desired outcome is a routine review and update, roles and responsibilities of the C-suite and board will be both time and scope limited and focused on ensuring appropriate progress and approval of next year's action plan developed by the management team.

3. *Context.* Appropriate context for the review and update must be established by some indication that the process is kicking off. Generally, if only minimal updating is in order, beginning the update can be accomplished via an informal meeting paired with written or electronic communication wherein desired outcomes and roles are explained. Expecting an extensive update, however, calls for a more formal kickoff with a broader audience and includes proposing a more structured update process, time line, and roles. Ensuring sufficient context also entails any preparatory activities related to gathering the performance

data required to conduct the review and identifying any additional data needed to support environmental assessment updates.

Process Options

In nearly all cases, the process used in the annual update will be far less extensive than that employed in the initial development of the strategic plan. However, it is hard to accurately assess the minimum necessary amount of work required to adequately update plans, and there are no hard-and-fast rules for this determination. Clearly, if a more robust update is called for, a more substantive process will be required. But even knowing this, what a "more substantive process" entails is subjective and depends on organizational dynamics and leadership preferences, among other factors. Thus there are almost unlimited options for what and whom to include in the process, and for how to approach and carry out the update. So as not to get overwhelmed by all of the process options available, the authors of this chapter have categorized process intensity into three points on a process-intensity continuum.

1. *Informal and very abbreviated process.* Even when a limited update is warranted, some attention should be paid to the outputs of each of the four strategic planning stages. Though this attention may be largely cursory in nature, affirming the continued relevancy of all key plan outputs is important; it is also vital to document doing so. If staying at the minimalist end of the process-intensity continuum makes sense, the work can typically be done by planning staff with oversight from a few senior leadership champions. These individuals assume responsibility for carrying out the review and update activities, with modest input or participation from others. Select input may be sought to validate the externally oriented portion

of the environmental assessment, specifically future environmental assumptions, and to identify any fine-tuning of major initiatives under way to address the critical planning issues. A summary of the review process and proposed modifications may be prepared and provided to additional members of the senior team or the planning committee for endorsement before commencing action planning for the following year.

2. *Formal but somewhat abbreviated process.* This option is likely best suited to situations such as scenario 3 in exhibit 10.1, wherein change has occurred or new environmental threats are looming, but overall direction, goals, and initiatives are still largely relevant. Completion of the update requires more senior management and staff effort, and more input and participation are needed. This process includes a more thorough update of the environmental assessment outputs to confirm that critical planning issues still reflect priorities. Adjustments to strategy formulation outputs—goals, metrics, major initiatives—are appropriate. To carry out these activities, a few structured review-and-update sessions should be held to get input and participation from a range of key internal stakeholders. Critical issue champions should spearhead these efforts, and the strategic planning committee should be engaged to review and affirm the changes proposed before passing along for C-suite or board approvals.

3. *Formal and lengthy update process.* Here, as in scenario 4 of exhibit 10.1, significant internal or external change has occurred, and more is likely to come. In these situations, the update process will involve a fairly hard look at the environment and assumptions about the future and may call for redefining the critical planning issues. As such, the products of strategy formulation—goals with metrics and major initiatives—will need thorough review and likely substantive modification. A review of organizational

direction—vision and overall strategy—should be undertaken and possibly tweaked. In proportion to the amount of update contemplated, input and participation from senior executives is needed, as is fairly extensive involvement of the strategic planning committee. It may be most effective to create task forces, overseen by key members of the strategic planning committee, charged with proposing changes to the results of the environmental assessment, strategy formulation, and organizational direction. Recommendations from the task forces should be formally presented to the entire planning committee, including C-suite leaders, for their feedback and decision making. The transition to developing action plans for the next year should also involve more extensive participation than typically necessary.

Many organizations have found that retreats (see chapter 4) are an excellent vehicle for accomplishing a significant portion of the input and participation called for in the annual strategic plan update. Obviously, the need for and desirability of retreats will vary some-what depending on the scope and extent of the update required. Nonetheless, a growing number of healthcare organizations have at least one annual strategic planning retreat as an important element of the annual update process.

Tips for Review and Update by Planning Stage

Environmental Assessment

Given that the inputs to this planning stage are indicative of the current state and emerging trends, the environmental assessment is likely to appear (and be) out-of-date most quickly. However, what matters most to the rest of the plan are the three main outputs of this stage—competitive advantages and disadvantages, future environmental assumptions, and critical planning issues. Therefore, while it is advisable to review and update the organizational performance and position information that drives these work products, doing so should be a focused activity. More specifically, the time and energy expended should be proportionate to the degree to which these input updates are likely to significantly affect the three main outputs. C. Davis Fogg (2010) suggests that, assuming the internal and external environment has not radically changed since plan completion, the environmental assessment should be "surgically updated." That is, the review and update should focus on the specific elements that have been affected by change and that are likely to affect the primary outputs.

Many provider organizations use national trend reports, such as *Futurescan: Healthcare Trends and Implications* (published annually by the Society for Healthcare Strategy & Market Development of the American Hospital Association and the American College of Healthcare Executives [ACHE]), to identify key shifts in the field and determine the degree to which these shifts are relevant and visible in their market and to their organization. Summaries of these types of materials also lend themselves well to kicking off the review and update process, as they can generate productive, high-level dialogue on trends with potentially critical strategic implications. Brief reviews of key local, regional, state, and national developments over the past year may also be helpful for staff to prepare, as may be a list of major organizational accomplishments. A structured discussion of these developments and of organizational accomplishments is recommended with the senior management team.

In circumstances of low to moderate change (scenarios 1 and 2), it is likely sufficient to review and tweak parts of the strength, weakness, opportunity, and threat (SWOT) analysis as appropriate, modify the list of future environmental assumptions as necessary, and affirm the critical planning issues. In circumstances of moderate to high change (scenarios 3 and 4), it is appropriate to revise the SWOT more fully, create a new list of future environmental assumptions, and revise existing critical issues to be more relevant, or to develop a revised list of critical planning issues. Whether the changes are minor or significant, reviewing them in a format that shows what has changed and what remains unchanged can help quickly clarify how the changes to the environmental assessment may point to necessary updates to goals, metrics, and initiatives.

Organizational Direction

Ordinarily, this component of the strategic plan requires the least attention in the annual update; organizational direction outputs should remain largely intact from update to update. The mission and values statements are the most timeless and least likely to require modification. Even in today's tumultuous environment, the vision and overall strategy should last at least five years for the majority of healthcare provider organizations.

Strategy Formulation

If the preliminary assessment responses align with scenarios 1 or 2 (see exhibit 10.1), the focus of reviewing and updating the strategy formulation is exclusively on examining progress related to the plan's goals and objectives. Revisions may be warranted because of actual implementation success or failure, including pace of progress, roadblocks encountered, and the like.

If the preliminary assessment responses align with scenarios 3 or 4, the review and updating of strategy formulation may be conducted in a manner similar to that followed in the complete planning process or, depending on current circumstances, in a less or more process-intensive fashion. Assuming new critical issues were identified in the update of the environmental assessment stage, new goals, metrics, and initiatives will need to be developed for these new critical issues. Even if critical issues remain largely the same, some updating of goals, metrics, and major initiatives should be carried out to account for the significant change since completion of the last plan. Similar to the environmental assessment, senior management, at minimum, discusses and reviews strategy. Typically, and if using a more process-intensive approach, the strategic planning committee is briefed and reviews the strategy formulation outcomes.

Implementation Planning

Regardless of how much updating has been done to the products of the other planning stages, this stage should entail development of a new action plan for the next year. Even if there are only minimal updates in the strategy formulation phase (scenarios 1 or 2), it is always necessary to update action plans to account for progress made and challenges encountered in the previous year. See "Approach" for scenarios 1 and 2 in exhibit 10.1 for detail on the types of updates to the implementation plan that are most applicable.

In the case of scenario 2, in which progress has been inadequate, this time is advantageous for making sure that accountability is focused on individuals as opposed to groups and that the right individuals are chosen. When individuals realize that their implementation performance will be reviewed, the culture of an organization can shift toward accomplishment of each step toward strategic goals and the organizational vision.

Significant strategy formulation output updates (scenarios 3 or 4) require developing a brand new action plan to identify new objectives for each goal and metric and to establish new tactics.

At the conclusion of the annual update, board approval of the new strategic plan may be required. The scope and extent of the changes to the plan ordinarily will dictate how involved the approval process needs to be. Even if the board does not need to approve the changes, organizations can increase board commitment to the planning process and organizational strategy by apprising the board of progress on the plan, and informing them when the plan has been actively and thoughtfully revised.

A Few Examples

Jefferson Health

Jefferson Health in Philadelphia, Pennsylvania, the clinical delivery system of Thomas Jefferson University, comprises Thomas Jefferson University Hospital, Abington Health, and Aria Health. The organization carries out its annual strategic plan updates as illustrated in exhibit 10.2. This process results in an annual update of its three-year rolling strategic plan. The strategic planning calendar is integrated with the organization's key operational and fiscal routines and staged over the course of the June fiscal year.

The annual strategic plan update begins in the summer, when management reviews the organization's progress against its plan for the previous year. At this time, it also assesses environmental changes and develops new or modified assumptions for the future. High-level system goals are also reviewed and revised as appropriate.

With these system parameters set, planning at the business unit and critical-issue level ensues over the next few months. Typically, teams for key service lines and organization-wide initiatives such as service excellence and quality or safety improvement develop detailed plans in each area. All of this effort rolls up to create the next version of the organization's strategic plan in December.

Following this phase, the plan presents issues to be considered during the budget development process and the annual operating plan in the latter half of the fiscal year. The results provide the balanced scorecard for use during the next fiscal year. Also, in the latter part of the fiscal year, research and information gathering, including surveys and data collection, are carried out to inform the plan update in the following fiscal year.

The processes of Ascension Health and the American College of Healthcare Executives both constitute useful examples.

Ascension Health

Ascension Health, a large St. Louis–based Catholic healthcare system, has an annual process called the Integrated Strategic, Operational, and Financial Plan (ISOFP) for the system and its members. The process formerly resulted in a five-year plan, but in 2015, given the dynamic nature of healthcare and rapid changes in the environment, Ascension Health converted to a three-year plan. However, it noted that the strategic horizon for the ISOFP should still be

Exhibit 10.2: Jefferson Health Planning Cycle

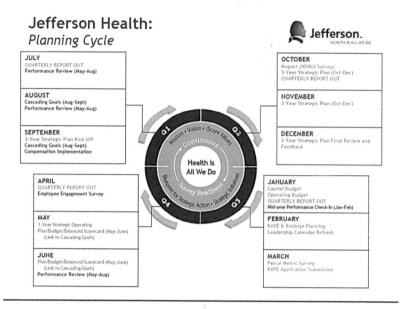

Jefferson Health:
Planning Cycle

Jefferson.
HEALTH IS ALL WE DO

JULY
QUARTERLY REPORT OUT
Performance Review (May-Aug)

AUGUST
Cascading Goals (Aug-Sept)
Performance Review (May-Aug)

SEPTEMBER
3-Year Strategic Plan Kick-Off
Cascading Goals (Aug-Sept)
Compensation Implementation

APRIL
QUARTERLY REPORT OUT
Employee Engagement Survey

MAY
1-Year Strategic Operating
Plan/Budget/Balanced Scorecard (May-June)
(Link to Cascading Goals)

JUNE
Plan/Budget/Balanced Scorecard (May-June)
(Link to Cascading Goals)
Performance Review (May-Aug)

OCTOBER
Magnet (NDNQI Survey)
3-Year Strategic Plan (Oct-Dec)
QUARTERLY REPORT OUT

NOVEMBER
3-Year Strategic Plan (Oct-Dec)

DECEMBER
3-Year Strategic Plan Final Review and
Feedback

JANUARY
Capital Budget
Operating Budget
QUARTERLY REPORT OUT
Mid-year Performance Check-In (Jan-Feb)

FEBRUARY
KAPE & Baldrige Planning
Leadership Calendar Refresh

MARCH
Pascal Metric Survey
KAPE Application Submission

Health Is All We Do — Q1 · Q2 · Q3 · Q4 — Mission · Vision · iScore Values · Continuous · Survey Readiness · Blueprint for Strategic Action · Strategic Initiatives

Source: Jefferson Health (2015). Used with permission.

five years, with a focus on those strategies that affect the fiscal year 2016–2018 operational and financial plans.

Strategic planning begins with reconsidering overall system direction, including Ascension Health's strategies, guiding principles, and key assumptions. Then, detailed planning occurs in the defined regions, called Ministry Markets, that Ascension services. Ascension Health provides strategic plan content and process guidance via a content guide that contains templates, process steps, and a schedule. The process at the regional level kicks off in December, about midway through Ascension Health's fiscal year.

Ministry Market leaders are provided with a content guide that

- promotes rigor, accountability, and consistency across each Ministry Market ISOFP;

- guides each Ministry Market on the strategic, operational, and financial content that should be in the ISOFP;
- helps Ministry Market leaders conduct meetings with Ascension Health leaders to review their annual ISOFP;
- provides a template for the ISOFP; and
- includes other resources to simplify the process.

As various parts of the ISOFP are drafted, a fairly intensive process of region-specific strategic and financial planning and regular interactions with system strategy and finance staff ensues over the next few months.

Each Ministry Market ISOFP addresses strategy, capital requirements, operational plans, and financial plans and budgets. Therefore, in each Ministry Market the ISOFP process is designed to involve clinical, finance, operational, strategy, and business development leadership. Ascension develops a full draft of each region's ISOFP by late March and, after reviews by system leadership, the regional plans are finalized by mid-April. Over the next two months, the plans are consolidated into an Ascension-wide plan and reviewed and approved by the office of the president, board committees, and board of directors.

American College of Healthcare Executives

ACHE has a long history of strategic planning and a well-developed annual update process. ACHE's most recent deep dive on its strategic plan was conducted in 2013–2014, resulting in the 2015–2017 ACHE Strategic Plan. Following this step, annual updates occur each year through the strategic planning process. In 2017 another deep dive will be conducted to develop the 2018–2020 ACHE Strategic Plan.

ACHE conducts a systematic annual planning process to develop and deploy its strategic plan using a four-step methodology:

1. Gather data and analyze
2. Develop plan attributes and initiatives

3. Operationalize the plan by deploying within the organization and with key partners
4. Execute, monitor, and adjust the plan as necessary

ACHE has four major initiatives supported by more specific tasks that guide the work plan toward achieving its defined goals and objectives. Each of the tasks is assigned to a specific executive or group to lead implementation. During the year, the organization monitors progress on these tasks quarterly and reports to the membership on the ACHE website.

Each year, executive staff formally review progress relative to plans and provides an update for next year's plan as required. In the past, updates to initiatives and tasks have been modest, absent dramatic changes in the environment. At a minimum, the annual updates will result in a revised set of tasks for each initiative for the following year. The board formally reviews the annual update before it is adopted. Once it is approved, implementation begins, progress is monitored and reported, and before long, the next annual update cycle commences.

Final Thoughts on the Review and Update Processes

An Art Not a Science

Unfortunately, how frequently a comprehensive strategic plan should be completed, relative to the less-intensive annual updates, depends on the organization, its environment, its particular circumstances, leadership style, cultural norms, and an array of other factors. In addition, as described earlier, even once it is determined that the update route is preferable, there is no "one-size-fits-all" approach that can be prescribed.

Fortunately, the growing insufficiency of annual updates is usually evident to organizations because the organization or its environment has changed markedly, the update process has started to become stale, the organization has largely accomplished (or has made substantial progress toward) key goals, or some combination of all three.

Integration Improves Effectiveness

The annual strategic plan update should be integrated with financial and operational planning to the extent possible. For most healthcare organizations, the annual update occurs during the first half of the fiscal year. When beginning an annual update process, many healthcare organizations erroneously delay the start (and completion) of the update process until later in the year and find that the necessary information for the budgeting process is not available in a timely manner. Experience indicates that an early start in the fiscal year provides for smoother integration with financial planning.

As a practical matter, the work flow needs to be staged and sequenced throughout the year, so that all elements of the management plans receive appropriate and thorough attention. Typically, the bulk of the work on the strategic plan update should be completed before financial and operating planning begins. However, some flexibility must be built into the process so revisions of all plans can be made as necessary before finalization, depending on the results of each element of this process. The third and (principally) fourth quarters can be used for iterative revisions to the strategic, financial, and operating plans.

Getting Perspective on the Role of the Update

The annual update should be treated as the mechanism and forum for formalizing appropriate adaptation, and it should be viewed as the component of broader strategic plan implementation that reconciles change over time. Inevitably, as implementation occurs, variation from what was envisioned will be called for and put into practice. Some of these ideas and opportunities may be so compelling or emergent that they are acted on before the next plan update occurs. Others may be held for consideration at the time of the update, though this delay is certainly not necessary. In either case, the annual update is the time and place to document these events and to test for their consistency with and relevance to the strategic plan.

REFERENCES

Fogg, C. D. 2010. *Team-Based Strategic Planning: A Complete Guide to Structuring, Facilitating, and Implementing the Process.* N. p.: CreateSpace Independent Publishing Platform.

Jefferson Health. 2015. Internal presentation. September 19.

Optimizing Strategic Planning

CHAPTER 11

Enabling More Effective Execution

Things don't just happen, they are made to happen.

—John F. Kennedy

To-morrow let us do or die.

—Thomas Campbell

THE CHALLENGES OF IMPLEMENTATION

Strategic planning has been criticized for its detachment from day-to-day operations and its inability to effect significant change in an organization. While comprehensive, well-designed plans may be prepared with exceptionally strong supporting documentation and the use of thorough, inclusive consensus-development processes, implementation seems to be elusive and ultimately out of reach for many organizations.

Implementation difficulties are not unique to healthcare organizations. According to Michael C. Mankins and Richard Steele (2005, 64), companies worldwide "typically realize only about 60 percent of their strategies' potential value because of deficits and breakdowns in planning and execution" (see exhibit 11.1). Farias Souza (2009) of the Balanced Scorecard Collaborative estimates that 90 percent of all companies fail to execute their strategies (see exhibit 11.2). A 2005–2006 study of the state of the art in healthcare strategic planning found that effectiveness of strategic plan implementation was rated relatively low by respondents, and the ability to handle curve balls and other new developments and adjust the plan and implementation was rated the lowest of all strategic planning skills and components (Zuckerman 2007).

Why is there such a high failure rate in the transition from planning to implementation? It appears to be a function of four main factors:

1. *Loss of energy and focus.* In many organizations, strategic planning is an event that engages a broad spectrum of leadership. It is a high-level, high-visibility process that garners considerable attention and effort. Once the strategic plan has been completed and approved, the show is over and implementation occurs in a much less public and celebrated manner. This loss of energy and focus may ultimately cause implementation to be inconsistent and to dissipate slowly over time.

2. *Lack of management.* As described later in the chapter, implementation needs to be actively managed. It does not just happen but rather requires a significant amount of hard work, direction, and oversight. Yet, in the aftermath of many strategic planning efforts, implementation is assumed to occur rather than be actively managed; in these cases, the implementation failure rate is high.

3. *Disconnect from operations.* Strategic planning is often viewed as an add-on to day-to-day operations; if done periodically, rather than in an ongoing manner, the fragmentation is aggravated. In these situations, the implementation plan does not belong to anyone and is not a part of anything that routinely occurs in operations. This disconnect makes it difficult to maintain a focus on implementation and regularly and consistently make progress.

Exhibit 11.1: Where the Performance Goes

This chart shows the average performance loss implied by the importance ratings that managers in our surgery gave to specific break-downs in the planning and execution process

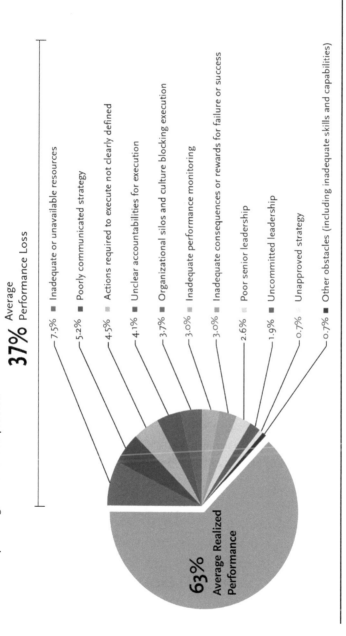

37% Average Performance Loss

- 7.5% ■ Inadequate or unavailable resources
- 5.2% ■ Poorly communicated strategy
- 4.5% ■ Actions required to execute not clearly defined
- 4.1% ■ Unclear accountabilities for execution
- 3.7% ■ Organizational silos and culture blocking execution
- 3.0% ■ Inadequate performance monitoring
- 3.0% ■ Inadequate consequences or rewards for failure or success
- 2.6% ■ Poor senior leadership
- 1.9% ■ Uncommitted leadership
- 0.7% ■ Unapproved strategy
- 0.7% ■ Other obstacles (including inadequate skills and capabilities)

63% Average Realized Performance

Source: Mankins and Steele (2005).

Exhibit 11.2: Four Barriers to Strategy Execution

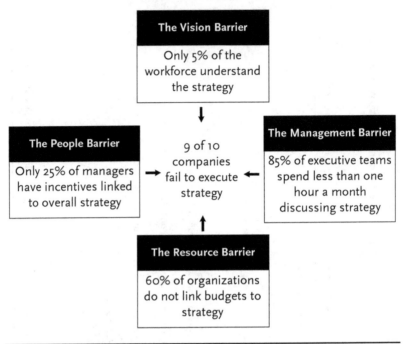

The Vision Barrier

Only 5% of the workforce understand the strategy

The People Barrier

Only 25% of managers have incentives linked to overall strategy

9 of 10 companies fail to execute strategy

The Management Barrier

85% of executive teams spend less than one hour a month discussing strategy

The Resource Barrier

60% of organizations do not link budgets to strategy

Source: Jefferson Health (2015).

4. *Lack of resources.* Many strategic plans are overly ambitious and unrealistic. They call for too many activities and actions to be implemented concurrently and devise strategies that exceed the organization's resources. Frustration emerges as it becomes clear that implementation is in jeopardy.

This chapter describes methods and processes to achieve a higher rate of implementation success; integrate strategic planning better into regular, ongoing organizational management; and ultimately evolve from the periodic strategic planning processes of the last several decades to the more effective and contemporary strategic management processes.

FOSTERING IMPLEMENTATION SUCCESS

Making a smooth, effective, and ultimately successful transition from planning to implementation starts with a sound, well-understood implementation plan. Many organizations display a tendency to rush into implementation at the conclusion of the strategic planning process and not prepare thorough, thoughtful implementation plans. In such plans, the roles and responsibilities of staff must be understood and accepted, as well as the time frame and interrelationships of implementation activities. Finally, and possibly foremost, a management structure and approach to implementation needs to be in place. The structure and approach must include, at minimum, a designated overall implementation leader and regular progress reviews. These reviews could involve senior management, corporate staff (in a system), or the strategic planning committee of the board. Effective implementation is a highly iterative process, so that review often leads to revision followed by subsequent implementation, further review, more revision, and so on, in a continuous cycle.

As discussed in Alan Zuckerman's 2005 article, "Executing Your Strategic Plan," and since redefined in this book, there are ten steps to successful plan implementation:

1. *Understand that plan execution starts during the preplanning.* The tone, content, and approach of an organization's strategic planning process all influence the likelihood of its success. Involve key stakeholders—board members, board planning committee members, physicians, other clinicians, senior and other managers, and planning staff. Communicate the importance of the strategic planning process, and make sure that everyone understands the benefits (community, financial, product or market, operational) of a well-executed plan. If you sought consulting assistance for development of the strategic

plan, consider retaining that assistance to monitor implementation.

2. *Consider execution while formulating strategy.* Execution is not something to worry about later; it must be an underlying theme during strategy formulation. However, execution worries should not dampen the creative spirit of strategy formulation. Instead, execution issues must be one of the many considerations of planning and doing that occur later in strategic planning. Think about whether high-level strategies can be subdivided into and executed at the operational level. You should be able to align individual actions with organizational strategies.

3. *Choose execution leaders wisely.* Having the right leaders with the right skills in place during plan execution can be the difference between success and failure. When you are selecting execution leaders, carefully consider skill level, ability to engender a sense of strategy ownership, and capacity for communicating. Ensure that leaders have the tools, resources, and training they need. More important, give them the time to finish the job—a chief complaint among execution leaders is a shortage of time. Last, make sure that leaders can resist the urge to meddle. When execution committees are managing implementation well, leaders need to know when to get out of the way.

4. *Mobilize the team and communicate.* Clarify roles and responsibilities of those involved in plan execution. In many organizations, there will be an oversight group of senior executives, leaders of individual initiatives and tasks, and supporting staff and groups. Make sure the implementation team is in place and clearly charged with carrying out its responsibilities as this phase begins.

5. *Mark the implementation phase in a formal, celebratory way.* As planning concludes and execution begins, organizations should select a formal approach for communicating

to their staff that implementation is beginning. Most important, plan an inclusive rollout event to show that the planning is complete and a new era is beginning. A celebratory occasion can help draw attention, raise expectations, and build enthusiasm that will be needed during implementation.

6. *Drive the plan down into the organization.* Strategy execution is most successful when it is seen as an organization-wide effort rather than an executive office exercise. Individuals throughout the organization must be given clear directions about what they are expected to achieve. Build implementation tasks into performance objectives and give rewards when they are completed. Using implementation subcommittees— with no more than 12 members—may help. Consider having these subcommittees in place during the strategic planning process, then transitioning them to a new role in implementation. All organizations may also need to provide training to individuals responsible for implementation.

7. *Watch out for the warning signs of execution failure.* Some common red flags that implementation is not progressing as it should include persistent political infighting, a loss of focus, a sense of inertia, pervasive resistance to change, and a disconnect between planning objectives and operational realities. If any of these issues crop up, quickly defuse the situation and aggressively pursue getting implementation back on track.

8. *Communicate, communicate, communicate.* Strategy execution involves even more people than strategy formulation, making communication crucial. Establish a common message about the strategic plan, make copies of the plan summary available, and provide web-based updates and internal communications via e-mail and other organizational media. The CEO and other senior managers

should meet with key stakeholders directly to provide feedback and respond to concerns.

9. *Have a monitoring system in place.* To track the implementation schedule, budget, and progress, use a monitoring system your organization finds relevant, accurate, and useful. Consider using a system that also measures the intangibles—management effectiveness, innovation, and potential for further progress. A good monitoring system will help you review the progress of the plan's implementation. The review should help organizations ensure that progress is being made, priorities stay on track, obstacles to progress are resolved, and resources are reallocated, if needed.

10. *Consider moving from strategic planning to strategic management.* Strategic planning is criticized for its detachment from day-to-day operations and its inability to produce real, sustainable change in organizations. Many organizations use strategic *management* approaches to integrate core management processes. Strategic management, discussed further later in this chapter, has clear benefits, such as integration (rather than coordination) with finance and operations and the fact that day-to-day management occurs in a strategic framework rather than in separate management processes. Organizations that use strategic management often find that their organizational culture starts adapting to change more easily.

ONGOING REVIEW OF PROGRESS

C. Davis Fogg (2010, 215) suggests that ongoing review of progress "helps you keep the plan on track once implementation is under way, reallocate resources as you accomplish goals or your strategic situation changes, imbed accountability for program accomplishment with every implementer, and reward results to ensure commitment and continued top level performance." He believes that the key to success is

- "review, review, review;
- revise, revise, revise; and
- reward, reward, reward."

There are five main reasons for conducting regular progress reviews:

1. To shine the spotlight on the ongoing importance of implementation to the organization's success
2. To encourage and motivate individuals and teams involved in implementing action plans through visibility, recognition, and praise
3. To make sure that appropriate progress is being made and that priorities stay on track
4. To discuss and resolve problems and internal obstacles to progress, particularly those that require interdisciplinary intervention
5. To allow reallocation of valuable resources to the areas that most need them

Both formal and informal mechanisms can be used to effectively review ongoing progress. Regular meetings of senior management or the strategic planning committee of the board are one common approach to this task. For many organizations, monthly progress review meetings for the first year or two after completion of a major strategic planning effort help ensure progress and accountability. Frequent progress review meetings are the best way to ensure that implementation occurs and that timely adjustments are made to individual action plans.

Once the organization has accepted a disciplined approach to implementation, meeting frequency may be reduced. Mature strategic planning organizations find that quarterly or, in some instances, semiannual progress review meetings are sufficient to keep implementation on track.

A structured approach to implementation progress reviews often yields the best results. Such structure involves taking action plan formats, such as those provided in chapter 9, and marking them up in advance of each meeting, charting expectations versus actual results, schedules, resource consumption, and so on (see exhibit 11.3). Many organizations use a red, yellow, and green light schema to facilitate review of progress relative to the plan at a glance. Explanations of variances from expectations should be provided. New issues or concerns, or those that transcend individual action plans, can be noted in a comments section. Recommendations for changes to the implementation plan should also be noted. These progress reports should be circulated to all progress meeting attendees in advance.

Key to making these meetings more effective is a structured approach to meeting conduct. An important consideration is allowing enough dialogue to occur about action plans and issues that require group attention while minimizing discussion about things that do not require group discussion. In the absence of such focus, progress review meetings tend to be overly long and have diminished effectiveness as a result. In other cases, the meetings are too short and perfunctory.

The meeting leader needs to carefully craft the agenda to balance competing concerns and needs, all in a time frame that is appropriate to the importance of the topics being discussed. Advance preparation and awareness of pitfalls in this process help ensure that the progress review meetings achieve the intended outcomes and are a highly effective mechanism for ongoing plan implementation support.

Individual performance reviews also can enhance the effectiveness of plan implementation. If the action plan objectives are built into individual performance objectives, these annual or semiannual reviews provide an opportunity to review progress and make adjustments with individuals responsible for implementation.

Informal progress reviews can and should occur on an ongoing basis. Contact among senior leadership, some of whom may have direct implementation responsibilities, and between senior leadership and other staff with implementation responsibilities, should be frequent in most organizations. Such regular contact provides yet another opportunity for periodic, but less formal, review of progress against plan.

Even with the active monitoring process outlined in the earlier section, senior management may need to intervene directly in implementation to keep initiatives on track. Fogg (2010) notes four types of interventions that may be required:

1. Counseling an individual or team, providing advice for dealing with problems or problematic team members
2. Exerting influence to remove obstacles or obtain the resources needed to move forward
3. Improving skills, such as through training or by enhancing functional expertise
4. Providing direction, especially to get an individual or group back on track

Rewards also play an important role in facilitating achievement of implementation tasks. Individual and group performance may both be rewarded, and rewards can be both financial and nonfinancial in nature. Psychological rewards, including publicity for achievements or effort, and recognition for winning organizational contests, can play a key role in motivating individuals and teams to make good progress in implementation.

THE BALANCED SCORECARD

The balanced scorecard is a tool to assist with ongoing progress monitoring and implementation. It is estimated that more than 50

Exhibit 11.3: Action Plan Progress Review Example

Objective	Leader	Performance Level			Status Update
		Threshold	Target	Superior	
1. Improve the level of patient/customer satisfaction with Community Health (a subsidiary)	DP	Have a combined patient/client satisfaction score average of 94	Have a combined patient/client satisfaction score average of 95	Have a combined patient/client satisfaction score average of 96	Patient satisfaction score is 95%
2. Achieve high level of patient satisfaction with medical center services as measured by inpatients, outpatients, emergency department, and physician practices	LG	Demonstrate improvement in the average scores of two of the satisfaction surveys	Demonstrate improvement in the average scores of three of the satisfaction surveys	Demonstrate improvement in the average scores of four of the satisfaction surveys	3rd Quarter 2013 patient satisfaction improved in all four areas: —Inpatients YTD: 87.7 (vs. 2012 score of 86.7) —Outpatients YTD: 93.4 (vs. 2012 score of 93.1) —Medical practices: 92.1 (vs. 2012 score of 91.9) —Emergency department: 89.1 (vs. 2012 score of 87.9)

(continued)

(continued from previous page)

3. Increase average patient satisfaction with services in Hunterdon Imaging Associates and Hunterdon Center for Surgery	NH	Increase average Press Ganey scores by .5	Increase average Press Ganey scores by 1	Increase average Press Ganey scores by 1.5	Third quarter combined average for Hunterdon Imaging Associates and Hunterdon Center for Surgery was 93 vs. 2012 average of 93.6.
4. Achieve high level of employee engagement	VK	Achieve 50th percentile "Engaged" ranking	Achieve 65th percentile "Engaged" ranking	Achieve 75th percentile "Engaged" ranking	Employee engagement survey has been finalized. Achieved 58th percentile for employee engagement.
5. Achieve high level of physician engagement	VK	Survey employed and independent physicians using engagement tool	Using results of survey, develop a plan to improve physician engagement	Implement at least one strategy to improve engagement	Physician engagement survey closed with a 44% participation rate. A plan to improve physician engagement is being developed.

Source: Hunterdon Healthcare System (2013).

percent of large US companies use a balanced scorecard (Balanced Scorecard Institute 2015). Developed in industry in the early 1990s by Robert S. Kaplan and David Norton, it is intended to supplement traditional performance measurement systems by tracking "financial results while simultaneously monitoring progress in building the capabilities and acquiring the intangible assets [organizations] would need for future growth" (Kaplan and Norton 1996a, 75). John R. Griffith and Jeffrey A. Alexander (2002) describe the balanced scorecard as an integrated set of measures, driven by the organization's vision and strategy, typically covering the following dimensions in healthcare organizations:

- *Financial.* Financial performance and management of resources (including intangible resources such as workforce capability and supplier relations)
- *Internal business processes.* Cost, quality, efficiency, and other characteristics of goods and services
- *Customer.* Measures of satisfaction, market share, and competitive position
- *Learning and growth.* Measures of the ability to respond to changes in technology, customer attitudes, and economic environment

The balanced scorecard complements financial measurements with measurements of progress in three key areas: customer satisfaction, internal business processes, and learning and growth (see exhibit 11.4). Improvements in the balanced scorecard approach have rendered it a valuable tool for some companies that have used it as a key part of a strategic management system (see next section). Kaplan and Norton (1996a, 75) suggest that "used this way, the scorecard addresses a serious deficiency in traditional management systems: their inability to link a company's long-term strategy with its short-term actions."

Exhibit 11.4: Translating Vision and Strategy: Four Perspectives

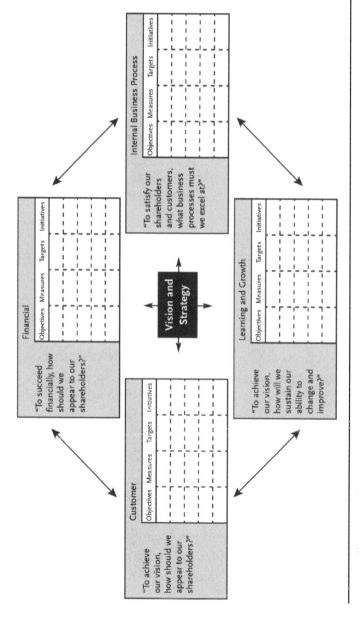

Source: Jefferson Health (2015).

A number of healthcare organizations have adopted the balanced scorecard as an aid in strategy implementation. Noorein Inamdar and Robert S. Kaplan (2002) cite five potential benefits of this approach for healthcare organizations:

1. It aligns the organization around a more market-oriented, customer-focused strategy.
2. It facilitates, monitors, and assesses the implementation of the strategy.
3. It provides a communication and collaboration mechanism.
4. It assigns accountability for performance at all levels of the organization.
5. It provides continual feedback on the strategy and promotes adjustments in response to marketplace and regulatory changes.

In a review of the literature on the use of the balanced scorecard in healthcare, Bob McDonald (2012) cites a few additional benefits of the balanced scorecard for healthcare organizations, including avoiding overemphasis on financial measures, enhancing focus on customer service, and improving outcomes.

In a review of the application of the balanced scorecard approach to healthcare organizations, Inamdar and Kaplan (2002) charted the steps involved in developing and implementing the balanced scorecard (see exhibit 11.5). Kaplan and Norton (1996a) suggest that the process of managing performance via the balanced scorecard consists of four sequential steps (see also exhibit 11.6):

1. *Translating the vision.* The mission and vision are often too abstract to be useful to employees as effective guides to day-to-day operations. Identifying concrete measures related to the mission and vision translates these lofty statements into a more effective form.

Exhibit 11.5: The Balanced Scorecard Development and Implementation Process

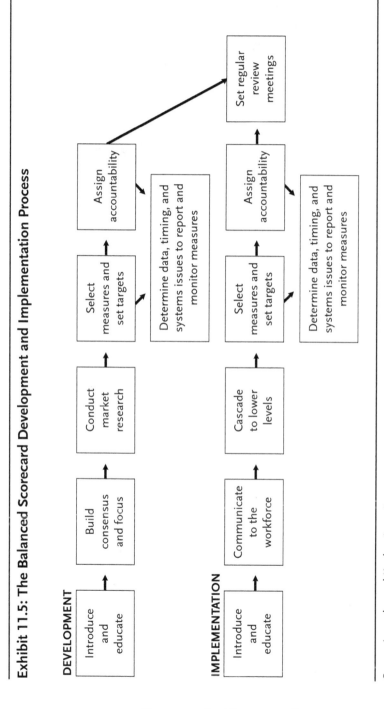

Source: Inamdar and Kaplan (2002).

Exhibit 11.6: Effectively Using the Balanced Scorecard to Manage Performance

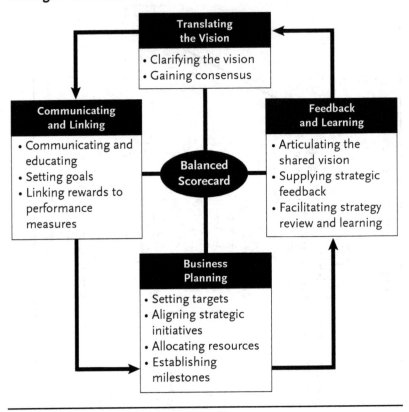

Source: Kaplan and Norton (1996b).

2. *Communicating and linking.* Involving employees from all levels of the organization in developing the scorecard initiates the process of integrating it into the organization. Ultimately, linking the scorecard measures to subgroup and individual performance measurements is the most effective approach.

3. *Business planning.* In this step, the overall strategy is translated into the objectives, measures, targets, and initiatives that link the strategy with operations and

implementation. Similarly, integration of strategic and budgeting or financial planning is inherent in the creation of the scorecard.

4. *Feedback and learning.* A balanced scorecard incorporates a process for review and evaluation of progress and modification of plans as necessary.

While using the balanced scorecard approach improves on previous performance measurement approaches, Kaplan and Norton (1996a, 85) argue that it is even more valuable "as the foundation of an integrated and iterative strategic management system." In these situations, companies are using the scorecard to

- clarify and update strategy,
- communicate strategy throughout the company,
- align unit and individual goals with the strategy,
- link strategic objectives to long-term targets and annual budgets,
- identify and align strategic initiatives, and
- conduct periodic performance reviews to learn about and improve strategy.

FROM STRATEGIC PLANNING TO STRATEGIC MANAGEMENT

Increasingly, healthcare organizations are moving beyond periodic strategic planning to more systematic approaches carried out regularly and integrated with other core management processes (see exhibit 11.7). Clear benefits may be derived in implementation rigor and implementation success. Also, the quality of strategic planning and implementation is improved as a result of better coordination with finance and operations in ongoing strategic planning processes. Additional benefits are obtained by those organizations that evolve to strategic management and integrate (rather than coordinate) finance and

Exhibit 11.7: Transitioning the Strategic Planning Process to Strategic Management

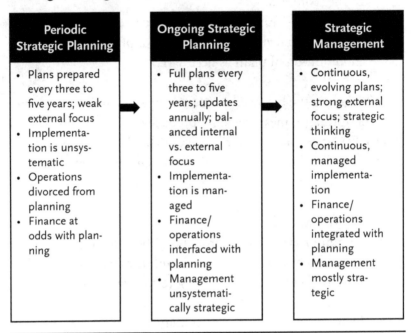

Periodic Strategic Planning	Ongoing Strategic Planning	Strategic Management
• Plans prepared every three to five years; weak external focus • Implementation is unsystematic • Operations divorced from planning • Finance at odds with planning	• Full plans every three to five years; updates annually; balanced internal vs. external focus • Implementation is managed • Finance/operations interfaced with planning • Management unsystematically strategic	• Continuous, evolving plans; strong external focus; strategic thinking • Continuous, managed implementation • Finance/operations integrated with planning • Management mostly strategic

operations with strategic planning as part of their regular management routines. Further, in strategic management, day-to-day management is carried out in a largely strategic framework, rather than the traditional separate management processes for operations, finance, and planning.

What exactly is strategic management? According to Denise Lindsey Wells (1996), it is (1) a systems approach to identifying and making necessary changes and measuring an organization's performance as it moves toward its vision, and (2) a management system that links strategic planning and decision making with the day-to-day business of operational management. Wells believes that planning is the prelude to strategic management. Strategic planning is insufficient if not followed by the development and implementation of the plan and evaluation of the plan in action.

The balanced scorecard is one proven approach to strategic management. Exhibit 11.8 presents another approach used by healthcare organizations. This approach is a logical extension of a strong strategic planning process transitioning into strategic management. Annually, three concurrent activities take place:

1. The strategic plan is developed or, following a comprehensive strategic planning process, updated in subsequent years. The plan update typically occurs in the first half of the fiscal year. In the second half of the year, planning initiatives provide inputs to capital and operating budgets and plans, and an iterative process leads to the finalization of all budgets and plans.

2. Throughout the year, implementation of the previously developed strategic plan occurs. This process is managed, with ongoing support and oversight of implementation—including formal review of progress and adjustment of implementation. Contingency plans for certain initiatives may be required.

3. Operations proceed routinely throughout the year. The implementation is managed within regular management structures and processes, and new strategic opportunities are reviewed and tested (with great frequency in some organizations) against the strategic plan. Such reviews may dictate adjustment of the plan's strategies and actions to accommodate new, emerging initiatives.

Whatever process organizations employ, strategic management represents a powerful tool with substantial benefits for both a stronger strategic planning function and a more successful implementation and integrated operations management function.

Exhibit 11.8: Annual Strategic Management Process Components

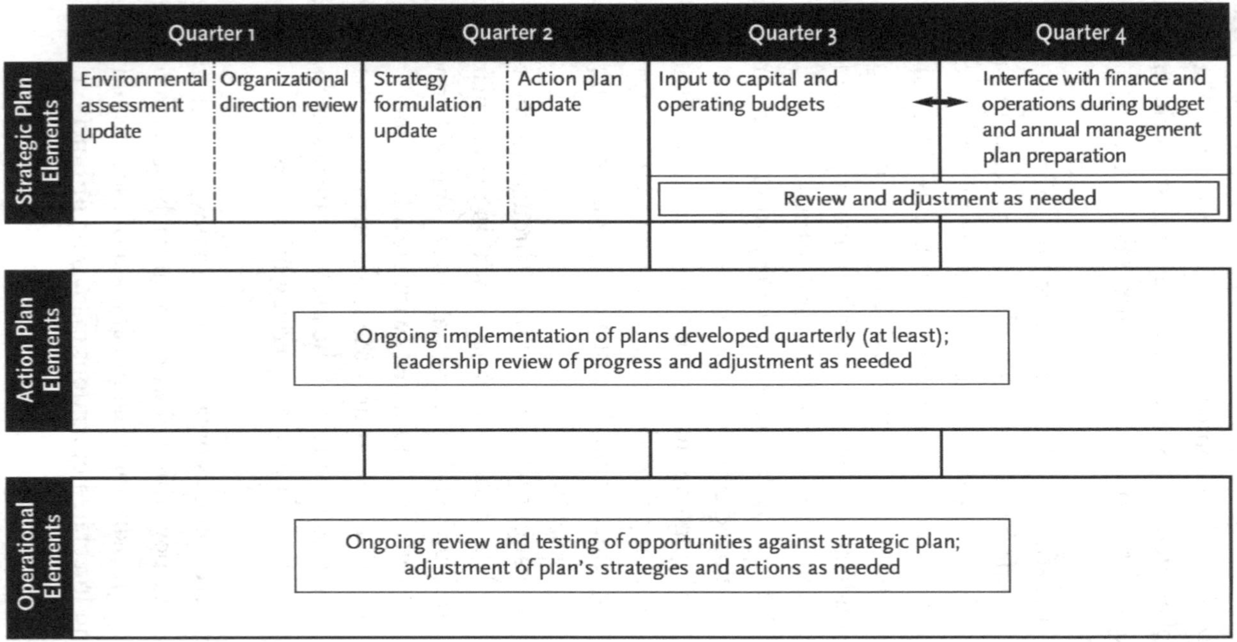

Strategic Plan Elements	Quarter 1	Quarter 2	Quarter 3	Quarter 4
	Environmental assessment update	Strategy formulation update	Input to capital and operating budgets	Interface with finance and operations during budget and annual management plan preparation
	Organizational direction review	Action plan update		
			Review and adjustment as needed	

Action Plan Elements
Ongoing implementation of plans developed quarterly (at least); leadership review of progress and adjustment as needed

Operational Elements
Ongoing review and testing of opportunities against strategic plan; adjustment of plan's strategies and actions as needed

© 2017 Veralon Partners Inc.

CONCLUSION

Effective implementation has proven to be difficult for most organizations. A common misperception is that implementation just happens, when in fact it must be carefully managed if the organization is going to meet its goals and objectives. Ongoing review of progress and new approaches, such as the balanced scorecard, should help keep implementation on track.

REFERENCES

Balanced Scorecard Institute. 2015. "Balanced Scorecard Basics." Accessed December 22. www.balancedscorecard.org/Resources/About-the-Balanced-Scorecard.

Fogg, C. D. 2010. *Team-Based Strategic Planning: A Complete Guide to Structuring, Facilitating, and Implementing the Process.* N. p.: CreateSpace Independent Publishing Platform.

Griffith, J. R., and J. A. Alexander. 2002. "Measuring Comparative Hospital Performance." *Journal of Healthcare Management* 47 (1): 42–43.

Hunterdon Healthcare System. 2013. Private correspondence. December 9.

Inamdar, N., and R. S. Kaplan. 2002. "Applying the Balanced Scorecard in Healthcare Provider Organizations." *Journal of Healthcare Management* 47 (3): 179–95.

Jefferson Health. 2015. Internal presentation. September 19.

Kaplan, R. S., and D. P. Norton. 1996a. *The Balanced Scorecard: Translating Strategy into Action.* Boston: Harvard Business Review Press.

———. 1996b. "Using the Balanced Scorecard as a Strategic Management System." *Harvard Business Review*, January–February, 75–85.

Mankins, M. C., and R. Steele. 2005. "Turning Great Strategy into Great Performance." *Harvard Business Review*, July–August, 64–72.

McDonald, B. 2012. "A Review of the Use of the Balanced Scorecard in Healthcare." Accessed December 31, 2015. www.bmcdconsulting.com/index_htm_files/Review%20of%20the%20Use%20of%20the%20Balanced%20Scorecard%20in%20Healthcare%20BMcD.pdf.

Souza, F. 2009. "An Introduction to the Balanced Scorecard and the Strategy Focus Organization." Balanced Scorecard Collaborative. Published March 6. www.slideshare.net/fariassouza/balanced-scorecard-collaborative-8491916.

Wells, D. L. 1996. *Strategic Management for Senior Leaders: A Handbook for Implementation.* Total Quality Leadership Office, Department of the Navy. Accessed January 11, 2017. http://govinfo.library.unt.edu/npr/initiati/mfr/managebk.pdf.

Zuckerman, A. M. 2007. *Raising the Bar: Best Practices for Healthcare Strategic Planning.* Chicago: Society for Healthcare Strategy & Market Development, American Hospital Association.

———. 2005. "Executing Your Strategic Plan." *H&HN Online.* Accessed January 11, 2012. www.hhnmag.com/hhnmag_app/jsp/artidedisplay.jsp?dcrpath=HHNMAG/PubsNewsArtide/data/050607HHN_Online_Zuckerman&domain=HHNMAG.

CHAPTER 12

Addressing Innovation in Strategic Planning

The greatest danger in times of turbulence is not the turbulence—it is to act with yesterday's logic.

—*Peter Drucker (attributed)*

The reasonable man adapts himself to the world: the unreasonable one persists in trying to adapt the world to himself. Therefore all progress depends on the unreasonable man.

—*George Bernard Shaw*

A fundamental component of the environmental assessment (see chapter 6) is anticipating and recognizing the implications of change in the market. This forecasting guides organizational direction (see chapter 7) and strategy formulation (see chapter 8). In considering likely changes, it is essential to distinguish between fads, which are short-term noise in the market, and major market shifts, which create new winners and losers. Some of those market shifts lead to game-changing innovations.

This chapter addresses two categories of innovation: (1) business model innovation, particularly related to alignment of providers and payers, and (2) clinical and technological innovation.

Business model innovation has had, and is expected to continue to exert, a dramatic impact on the economic alignment of providers with each other and with payers, while clinical and technological innovations have had and will have similarly significant impacts on access to and forms of wellness, as well as diagnostic and therapeutic care. Increasingly, both types of innovation are game changers rather than fads. Both have demonstrated the ability to improve value, defined as health outcomes achieved per dollar spent (Porter and Teisberg 2006), as well as the patient experience. As both types of innovation are expected to continue to alter profoundly the care model, the role of providers, and where care is provided, it is critical that they both be addressed in the strategic planning process.

Capitalizing on innovation can create new opportunities and competitive advantages. Conversely, when a healthcare organization ignores innovation during planning, a significant chance arises that it will miss a key opportunity or threat. Planners must include innovation in strategic planning, but they will find addressing it a challenge. Because innovation extends into areas that are less familiar issues for healthcare organizations, it warrants special attention.

Aligning the value sought by consumers (patients, employers, payers) with the value delivered by providers will increasingly be central to how healthcare organizations differentiate themselves and position themselves competitively. Because business model innovation and clinical and technologic innovation inform value, this chapter addresses topics related to the value equation in many of the planning steps. The value equation is

$$Value = (Quality + Patient\ Experience) / Price,$$

where *patient experience* is the aggregate of access, care coordination, and satisfaction.

INNOVATION IS OFTEN POORLY ADDRESSED

Healthcare organizations are often slow to recognize the potentially transformational impact of market changes. Some of this hesitation is natural, ingrained reluctance to move from successful strategies to new ones.

While incremental change is typically addressed in planning, many aspects of business model innovation and technological innovation are not. Among the reasons are the following:

- Fear that a particular innovation is just a fad
- Sectorwide attitude of risk aversion and insularity, combined with the viewpoint that healthcare is so unusual that changes that affect other fields are irrelevant
- Overconfidence in expert knowledge, to the exclusion of the customer's viewpoint
- Need to focus limited resources (people, time, funds) on resolving immediate challenges (e.g., maximizing fee-for-service revenue, reducing costs, strengthening physician alignment, forming strategic alliances)

CHANGE THAT MANDATES ACTION

The pace of change in the healthcare market continues to accelerate. As a result, markets are more competitive than in the past, with key barriers to competition disappearing (Harris and Frazier 2015).

To understand how innovation will affect strategy, we examine some of the changes that are driving a more competitive marketplace for healthcare services: the rise of consumerism, competition based on value, and the decline of geographic isolation.

Rise of consumerism. Armed with better information, emboldened through their experience in other industries, and with more convenient options now available to them, consumers are making their own healthcare choices. High-deductible health plans are encouraging individuals to shop for and act on price differentials for similar services (which were formerly masked by insurance benefits). In addition, the technology-based disruption that first took root in other sectors (e.g., online scheduling, mobile banking) has arrived in healthcare.

Competition based on value. As discussed earlier, payers (including Medicare) are beginning to reward providers that manage the total cost of care while maintaining or improving quality, patient experience, and access to care. Insurance products with narrow networks are often lower cost and attractive to individuals on insurance exchanges, adding to competition that affects provider market share. Differential copayments and deductibles, as well as convenience, steer patients to lower-cost settings for comparable services.

Decline of geographic isolation. Some hospitals and physicians have been the sole source of care in particular communities. As a result, they enjoyed monopoly pricing. Though some services will remain local, the same Internet technologies that are connecting individuals across the world are breaking into healthcare, reducing the power of local providers, who face competition from remote providers connecting with patients through video and other communication tools.

The shift toward a more competitive and dynamic market has enticed investors to support entrepreneurs pursuing clinical or technological and business model innovations that seek dramatic change in an inefficient system. These new entities hope to become new health sector powerhouses.

Proactive adoption of selected forms of innovation will help address three strategic imperatives for all healthcare providers. First, by its nature, innovation reinforces a focus on the future—anticipating and preparing for pending change. Second, it can enhance the value an organization delivers, enabling differentiation and improving market position. Third, it can create opportunities to improve financial performance.

Given the near-term priorities discussed earlier, as well as limited resources, few healthcare organizations have the ability to tackle more than a handful of the opportunities innovation presents. Thus, as with every other aspect of strategic planning, innovation opportunities must be prioritized and then staged over time: short-term (one to three years), intermediate (four to seven years), and long-term (eight years and beyond).

Bansi Nagji and Geoff Tuff (2012) describe a helpful approach to categorizing and prioritizing innovations. The Innovation Ambition Matrix in exhibit 12.1 allows a planner to plot innovations based on the degree to which they serve existing or new customers (y axis) and existing or new services (x axis). The result is three levels of innovation: core, adjacent, or transformational. Core innovations represent refinements to existing products and services for existing customers (e.g., new packaging for existing services), are typically handled in operating units of organizations, and depend on thoughtful analysis of straightforward market and organizational data. Adjacent innovations build on an organization's strengths, offering new services to a loyal customer base or offering a strong service to new customers. Transformational innovations involve providing new services to new markets. Such innovations often require establishing a new division—and teams with different expertise—to develop, launch, and deliver the new service or product.

In their research on industrial, consumer product, and technology companies, Nagji and Tuff suggest that the mix of innovations that led to better performance was 70 percent core, 20 percent adjacent, and 10 percent transformational. However, when they considered the returns on innovation investment, the results were flipped, with transformational innovation accounting for 70 percent of the returns, adjacent for 20 percent, and core innovation accounting for 10 percent of the returns. In other words, an overly conservative approach is likely to miss important opportunities. The applicability of these results to the healthcare sector must be considered. Given that healthcare providers have been relatively

Exhibit 12.1: The Innovation Ambition Matrix

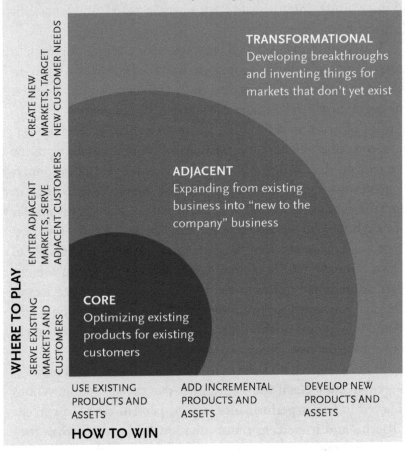

THE INNOVATION AMBITION MATRIX

Firms that excel at total innovation management simultaneously invest at three levels of ambition, carefully managing the balance among them.

WHERE TO PLAY

CREATE NEW MARKETS, TARGET NEW CUSTOMER NEEDS

ENTER ADJACENT MARKETS, SERVE ADJACENT CUSTOMERS

SERVE EXISTING MARKETS AND CUSTOMERS

TRANSFORMATIONAL
Developing breakthroughs and inventing things for markets that don't yet exist

ADJACENT
Expanding from existing business into "new to the company" business

CORE
Optimizing existing products for existing customers

USE EXISTING PRODUCTS AND ASSETS

ADD INCREMENTAL PRODUCTS AND ASSETS

DEVELOP NEW PRODUCTS AND ASSETS

HOW TO WIN

Source: Nagji and Tuff (2012).

258 *Healthcare Strategic Planning*

risk averse, some investment in transformational innovations is probably warranted.

This chapter provides a roadmap to addressing innovation in each step of the planning process—from environmental assessment to setting strategic direction, formulating strategy, and implementing—to enable healthcare organizations to successfully innovate. Because business model innovation differs from clinical and technological innovation, the approach to integrating each type of innovation into strategic planning is addressed separately in this chapter.

BUSINESS MODEL INNOVATION

To tackle the new competitive and financial drivers described earlier, healthcare providers are shifting their perspective and strategies to address consumerism and the total cost of care. A variety of labels have been used to describe business model innovations that align providers and payers, including *population health management, the shift from volume to value, risk-sharing, value-based contracting*, and *accountable care*.

Because health systems (including single-hospital organizations) are strong incumbents in healthcare delivery, they are at the center of much of this transformation. This section is therefore focused on the challenges and opportunities faced by health systems, though these challenges also apply to healthcare organizations throughout the continuum of care.

Addressing business model innovation in a strategic plan can be daunting and complex. Innovative business model strategies for health systems might include shifting payer contracting from volume to value, setting up new organizational structures to better coordinate care, or extending a provider's role to include insurance as well. This section provides a context and basic structure for those considerations.

The first step many health systems take in addressing business model innovation is to begin shifting payer contracting from a strictly fee-for-service basis to include more value-based payments based on quality and other performance measures. This shift should not only include managed care contract experts in the finance department. Shifting to value-based payment models (bundled payments, shared savings, risk sharing) requires a multidisciplinary effort, including physicians and leadership from finance, nursing care management, quality, and information technology.

A more intensive effort to shift from volume to value may involve setting up new organizational structures to better coordinate care. A clinically integrated network (CIN), accountable care organization (ACO), physician–hospital organization (PHO), or another multiprovider network typically engages independent physicians, along with hospital-employed physicians and health system leadership, in a joint structure created to drive improvement in quality and cost-effectiveness. Because these organizations have the power to define standards, contract with payers, and distribute shared savings or incentives from payer contracts, they represent strategic initiatives that must be designed thoughtfully with appropriate legal counsel. Some hospitals or health systems may have existing structures, in which case the task may be to revitalize an existing PHO or CIN rather than to create a new one.

Some health systems believe that they can best serve their communities and secure their market position by expanding vertically from healthcare delivery to insurance. This strategic initiative requires significant investment in start-up expenses and capital reserves, as well as new expertise not typically found in health systems.

ADDRESSING BUSINESS MODEL INNOVATION IN THE STRATEGIC PLANNING PROCESS

The following sections highlight how key issues related to business model innovation can be addressed in each step of the strategic planning process.

Environmental Assessment: External

The external environmental assessment should thoroughly identify the array of business model innovations taking place, the pace of change, and the implications of each of the following:

- Arrangements between competing providers and payers that can shift market share, either with narrow-network insurance products or value-based payment models
- New alignment models among providers in the market (e.g., clinically integrated networks, preferred networks for post-acute care) affecting relationships between physicians, health systems, and other provider organizations, and the ways in which these models are shifting referral relationships
- Emergence of nontraditional competitors, particularly those who engage patients earlier in the care process and could steer referrals away (e.g., clinics in big-box stores or retail pharmacy chains, smartphone-based services)
- Impact of Medicare payment models, which can add critical mass to population health initiatives
- Payer–provider innovations that over time may extend from more advanced markets to the local market

Environmental Assessment: Internal

In assessing their internal capabilities, providers must evaluate how well prepared they are to succeed in a field in which new business models are emerging. First, providers must honestly evaluate their current ability to manage for value—delivering patient care at the right time, in the right place, for the right cost. This evaluation requires determining the following:

- How far primary care physicians have come from a focus on "sick patient visits" to one based on keeping patients well—including those who don't come into the office
- How effective primary care physicians and those monitoring chronic conditions are at keeping patients out of the emergency department
- How effective patient transitions between units in the hospital and from the hospital to other care delivery sites (e.g., patient home or nursing facility) are, and the quality of related communications and monitoring (because transitions create patient vulnerability)
- How ready information technology (IT) and other infrastructure services are to support care and quality management
- How effectively the organization uses its electronic health records and data systems to support care management
- Whether the organization is positioned to measure and report key metrics such as quality of care, patient outcomes, patient satisfaction, and physician performance
- How well clinicians keep patients engaged

However, having these capabilities may not be enough to succeed. If the organization lacks sufficient scale to pursue required business model innovations, it may need to consider a merger or affiliation to increase the number of lives managed, the ability to diversify risk, the breadth of services offered, and geographic coverage.

Furthermore, the organization's pricing relative to competitors could also affect its ability to succeed in value-based contracts. If negotiated rates are higher than competitors' rates for similar services, market share may be at risk. If negotiated rates are lower, there may be an opportunity to grow market share and revenue.

Once the external and internal environments have been assessed and the summary of strengths, weaknesses, opportunities, and threats has been developed with business model innovations in mind, the organization needs to identify critical strategic issues to be addressed in the strategic direction phase of planning.

Organizational Direction

Setting organizational direction while taking account of business model innovation requires that the healthcare organization reevaluate mission and vision—the reasons the organization exists and what it seeks to achieve. Questions to be resolved include the following:

- What degree of financial risk does the organization want to accept for patient care?
- Is the organization interested in incorporating both provider and payer roles?
- In what parts of the continuum of care does the organization intend to have a role (e.g., wellness, ambulatory care, acute care, post-acute care)?
- Is the organization in the business of caring for the sick or improving or maintaining population health—or both?
- Must the organization own all aspects of the care in which it is involved, or is it willing to enter into strategic relationships with others to provide components of that care?

Strategy Formulation

In formulating strategies for business model innovations, healthcare organizations need to identify the specific business model innovations that may support their chosen strategic direction (e.g., form a CIN, launch an insurance business). When evaluating specific innovations, the planning team must engage finance leadership for the required financial modeling that helps determine whether the innovative business model strategies are economically viable. Unlike traditional strategic initiatives in which investment in services leads to additional volume and revenue, investment in value-based initiatives may lead to reductions in utilization rates and therefore reduced volume and possibly revenue. The chief financial officers of traditional providers often voice their concern that such initiatives will harm the volume-based bottom line. The analytic process should provide insight on such issues as the following:

- Whether market share can be increased or leakage reduced sufficiently to offset volume reductions from managing utilization
- How much volume would likely be lost if the organization does not pursue new business models as patients are steered to more efficient providers (opportunity cost)
- Whether investing in a CIN or other model can be more cost-effective than hospital employment to engage independent physicians
- What start-up investment and financial reserves are required, and what the range of financial burden might be

With a clear sense of financial opportunity and risk, it is helpful to determine whether partners are needed to develop the required infrastructure or provider network, establish the needed geographic coverage, and diversify risk. For example, even when they are successful, insurance divisions can be challenging to capital budgets, as successfully increasing enrollment results in additional required financial reserves that compete with traditional provider capital budgeting priorities for physical plant, equipment, and IT. Having completed these analyses, the planning team is able to determine which business model innovations should be included to support the goals and vision.

Implementation Planning

Because implementation of innovative business models requires skills that provider organizations may not already possess, the rollout of those models demands a special focus on acquiring the needed skills and expertise. Thus, in addition to more traditional tasks, implementation planning must include the following:

- Determining what skills will be obtained through training, recruitment, and partnering with other entities
- Specifying where revised role descriptions, performance review criteria, incentives, and progress tracking are required and who will be responsible for each of these
- Defining accountability processes specific to the innovation
- Identifying what education the board of directors may need to oversee these value-based business models, particularly where risk contracting or insurance is involved
- Specifying where independent physicians need to be engaged (e.g., independent physicians are typically involved in CINs as both participants and in governance) and how that will be achieved

Business model innovations may be pursued as an exciting opportunity or a defensive necessity. In either case, they are major strategic issues, or components of strategic issues, that require special attention during the strategic planning process (as described earlier).

CLINICAL AND TECHNOLOGICAL INNOVATION

The nature of clinical and technological innovation in healthcare is changing. While in previous decades most innovation sprang from large medical device and pharmaceutical companies and occurred in a framework of maximizing fee-for-service revenue, an increasing proportion of today's innovation is generated by entrepreneurs focused on increasing value in a market moving to fee-for-value. The innovator may be an "intrapreneur" at a big data or mobile phone company, but is just as likely to be an individual clinician or a small entrepreneurial firm. A huge pool of funds is available for investment, and venture capital and private equity firms see innovation in healthcare as having great potential for return on investment.

Several forces have long affected investments in clinical and technological innovation and will continue to do so. The Food and Drug Administration philosophy and approach to approvals for new devices, equipment, and drugs has a significant effect on innovation. Decisions by the Centers for Medicare & Medicaid Services (CMS) to pay for new technology, and CMS policy on whether it negotiates pharmaceutical pricing, further affects the attractiveness of investing in innovation. Finally, the overall investment environment and availability of capital for innovation across all sectors, and the relative attractiveness of the healthcare sector, determines how much capital is available for healthcare innovation.

In addition to these long-standing determinants of healthcare investment, some new dynamics have affected investment through 2016. The shift in focus from volume to value has created a new arena for investment. Investors look at the vast waste in the current delivery system and seek to finance clinical and technological innovations that will earn them a share of the savings, rather than just a fee for a unit of service. When this market environment is combined with the advancement of smartphone technology and communications infrastructure, a wide array of applications and wearables have found ready investors.

In this environment, many provider organizations see opportunities for their own innovations, or those of individual clinicians (e.g., physicians, nurses) that they employ. Some academic medical centers and health systems have set up incubators to attract entrepreneurial and creative clinicians and to help commercialize their innovations. This focus on innovation marks a broadening of the traditional academic medical center focus on research.

Clinical and technological innovation must be addressed in strategic planning because it will have a significant influence on the future of healthcare. Each innovation has the potential to have one or more of these six strategic impacts:

1. Enhancing the organization's ability to deliver better *value* by lowering costs and improving quality of clinical care, patient satisfaction, and access
2. Strengthening differentiation and positioning
3. Increasing the pace of the evolution of the *care delivery model* by more closely aligning providers and increasing the degree to which they accept risk (e.g., bundled payment, patient-centered medical homes, clinical integration, accountable care)
4. Shifting the *location of care delivery* from hospital campuses and long-term care facilities to new, lower-cost community-based care delivery sites (e.g., urgent care centers, retail and employer-based clinics, freestanding physician kiosks) and patients' residences (e.g., hospital at home, remote monitoring)
5. Changing the *provider team and its roles*, whether by modifying the required team composition (e.g., physicians, physician assistants, nurse practitioners, technicians, nutritionists, behavioral health providers) or the roles of team members (i.e., diagnostics, therapeutics, monitoring, wellness coaching)
6. Affecting the *ability of the organization to remain independent* or form alliances and partnerships rather than merging

There are currently five main types of clinical and technological innovation: clinical treatment, diagnostics, smart devices, telehealth, and predictive analytics. Exhibit 12.2 presents examples of each. By the time readers encounter this book, some of these may be in widespread use and others may have faded from view, replaced by the next wave of concepts and products. Proactively monitoring of new developments and considering how they may affect opportunities and market competition is critical.

To properly evaluate the merit of investing in or implementing individual clinical and technological innovations, such as those in the exhibit 12.2, planning teams should consider the associated impact on value. These examples illustrate the utility of doing so.

Exhibit 12.2: Types of Clinical and Technological Innovation

Type of Innovation	Examples of Innovation
Clinical treatment	• Implantation of computer-assisted sensory devices (i.e., retina, hearing) • Artificial tissues, fluids, organs • Bionic limbs • Exoskeletons • 3-D printing of bones, tissues, organs • Cellular-level therapies • Molecular-level therapies, including genetics
Diagnostics	• Lab tests with molecular-level diagnostics • Portable devices—point-of-care blood analyzers, hand-held ultrasound • Ingestible monitors for gastrointestinal visualization • Smartphone attachments (e.g., otoscopes, dermatoscopes, electrocardiograms [EKGs])
Smart devices	• Wearable monitors • Wristbands • Smart clothing (e.g., bras, socks, shirts, headbands, slippers) for tracking heart rate, blood pressure, temperature, and so on • Contact lens devices to measure blood glucose on an ongoing basis for people with diabetes • Transparent skin patches

(continued)

(continued from previous page)

Telehealth	• Patient portals for electronic visits with physicians, including second opinions and consultations • Video-based teleconsults between physicians • Remote interpretation and monitoring of imaging and EKG results and patient management (teleradiology, electronic intensive care units) • Physician kiosks at employer sites, retail stores, airports, libraries, and so on
Predictive analytics	• Evidence-based protocols based on large clinical datasets and powerful computer analytics • Aggregation of diagnostic data for use in predictive analytics and personalized care planning • Electronic health records with real-time diagnostic support • Clinician training based on computer-determined best practices • Risk-adjusted care management • Genomics and personalized care

Example 1: Three-Dimensional Printing (Also Known as Additive Manufacturing)

Three-dimensional printing—as the term is used in healthcare—refers to a process of recreating a physiological object through the successive layering of organic material via a computer-controlled process. Currently it is being applied to the formation of bones (e.g., jawbones, fingers, toes, vertebrae), bionic ears, facial prostheses (e.g., noses), and other items that are in turn implanted in patients. Work is under way to perfect the 3-D creation of human kidneys, livers, lungs, and hearts. Three-dimensional printing of tissues is based on highly biocompatible materials or even the patient's own stem cells.

This innovation has the potential to improve the transplant process in a number of ways. Patients who need transplants have historically had to endure long waits for a limited number of viable, tissue-matched organs, and after surgery, patients have received fairly intensive ongoing care at high cost. Generating new body parts would increase the precision while also reducing wait times and minimizing the odds of tissue infection and rejection. Together, these features could contribute to lowering the cost of treatment and enhancing the ability of the patient to resume a normal lifestyle, potentially adding value for risk-bearing providers.

Example 2: Remote Monitoring Devices

Remote monitoring devices allow an individual to monitor her own physiological health and transmit the data directly to clinicians without traveling to the physician's office, emergency department, or other setting. These devices enable clinicians to monitor patients remotely, supporting bedside testing in an acute, post-acute, or residential setting. They advance the use of the hospital-at-home concept, through which patients may be discharged quickly from an acute care setting and cared for in their homes.

The devices also enable early detection of problems, so that intervention can occur before acuity and cost of care increase. This is particularly helpful for patients with chronic illness (e.g., congestive heart failure, chronic obstructive pulmonary disease, diabetes), allowing wins on bundled payment programs or programs in which providers are at risk for the care quality and cost for a population. In these ways, the use of remote monitoring devices can be expected to contribute to changing the role of clinicians.

Example 3: Physician Kiosks

Physician kiosks use both telehealth and portable diagnostic technology to improve access to care and have been installed in retail pharmacies, shopping malls, workplaces, libraries, schools, airports, and other service locations. With an attendant's help and clinician direction, the patient interacts with a physician or advanced practice clinician via videoconferencing, using specific diagnostic equipment available in the kiosk. The equipment transmits results directly to the physician or other clinician.

Kiosks may be located in retirement communities to serve a concentration of patients with chronic conditions without requiring them to travel. It could allow a single clinician to serve patients in multiple locations in rapid succession. Because some patients would likely use kiosks instead of the emergency department or a physician's office, the kiosks could contribute to a reduction in population health costs.

ADDRESSING CLINICAL AND TECHNOLOGICAL INNOVATION IN THE STRATEGIC PLANNING PROCESS

Clinical and technological innovations can transform the role of the clinician, the location of care, and the nature of services provided by hospitals, physicians, and others. Given the magnitude of potential impacts innovation, it is vital that the planning process directly address the forms of change. The following sections highlight the key issues and questions related to clinical and technological innovation to explore in each step of the strategic planning process and tasks that should be applied in those steps.

Environmental Assessment: External

During the external environmental assessment, healthcare organizations should profile the stage of evolution of clinical and technological innovation both nationally and in their service areas, identifying innovations that are currently present or in the process of development. The planning team should complete the following four tasks as part of the environmental assessment:

1. Obtain the perspective of selected members of the clinical staff through individual and group interviews.
2. Review which innovations are being pursued by which competitors, as these may affect your competitive position.
3. Investigate whether community residents, payers, or employers are using, supporting, or advocating for any forms of technological innovation.
4. Finally, incorporate insights from journals, blogs, online discussion boards, and websites devoted to innovation and entrepreneurial activity, which should be monitored on an ongoing basis.

Once the profile is assembled, the organization should screen the innovations identified, assessing the following:

- Whether the form (or forms) of innovation appears to be a fad or is more likely to last and have a meaningful impact
- The extent to which the innovation is taking hold in the service area
- What innovations competitors are pursuing, and their likely impact on competitive position

This external assessment helps identify clinical and technological innovations that planning teams need to include for further consideration. Some innovations can be immediately ruled out, while others can be assessed in greater depth during strategy formulation. Furthermore, some innovations may not rise to the level of strategic decisions, while others may be strategic because of their potential to change an organization's position or because of the capital investment required.

Environmental Assessment: Internal

During the internal assessment, the organization should identify its own strengths and weaknesses as an innovator to determine the types of innovation that fit the organization's culture and business needs. The organization should

- assess current organizational capabilities to support clinical and technological innovation;
- examine the healthcare organization's history as a pioneer, early adopter, or lingerer at the trailing edge of innovation;
- identify innovators in the organization and their desire and ability to support future innovation;
- evaluate resources for technology transfer if innovations may return value to the organization; and
- consider whether pursuit of one or more of these forms of innovation will enable creation of compelling value equations.

If the internal or external assessments indicate that a particular innovation will have a significant effect on one of the six key strategic impacts listed earlier in the chapter (i.e., enhance value, differentiate, improve the care delivery model, shift the location of care, adjust the provider team, address independence vs. partnership), it should be addressed further in the stage of planning that addresses strategic direction. If it is not expected to have this effect, it should be moved to the sideline for further monitoring and reconsideration at a later point.

Organizational Direction

In formulating future direction, healthcare organizations must address how emerging clinical and technological innovations influence and are addressed in their mission, vision, and values statements and their overall organizational direction. Among the questions to be explored are the following:

- Whether the organization aspires to be a pioneer, early adopter, or follower of proven forms of technology
- How the organization's willingness to adopt innovation affects its focus on treating the sick and injured versus managing population health, and on its purpose as a leader in the delivery of clinical services, patient experience, or clinician training
- How the organization's adoption of clinical and technological innovation affects the desired state of the organization ten or more years in the future (its vision)

In assessing the impact of innovation on the vision, several factors should be considered, including the population served by the organization (e.g., health status issues addressed, patient acuity, geography); the breadth of the care continuum it provides; service delivery locations; and whether the organization will stand alone or partner with other providers, payers, retail organizations, or innovation companies of various types. The planning team should then determine whether and where clinical and technological innovation fits in the overall strategic direction of the organization.

Strategy Formulation

In formulating strategy, it is tempting but ill-advised to avoid innovation because it seems risky, unknown, and costly. Look more deeply to identify the strategic and operational significance and impact. Decisions to pursue innovations strategies should be based on a strong business case, not simply because they are the pet projects of notable individuals within the organization.

During the strategy formulation activity of strategic planning, clinical and technological innovations may fit as major or supporting initiatives. Therefore, include potential innovations among the strategies and initiatives considered to address the critical issues and to support fulfillment of the goals. As described in chapter 8, internal task forces may help to evaluate options and should be educated about the innovation options. It may be helpful to review the array of potential types of innovation (exhibit 12.2).

If innovations appear to support the goals, they should be analyzed and prioritized in the same way as other major initiatives and supporting initiatives. Because they often encompass more uncertainty, it may be helpful as well to categorize innovations as core, adjacent, or transformational (as described in exhibit 12.1).

Implementation Planning

Innovations can present certain unique considerations when shifting from strategy development to implementation. If the innovation is still being refined and is not fully ready to be applied, additional research, design, packaging, and other steps may be necessary. In that situation, the healthcare organization should designate an action step that takes the product or concept to an incubator or innovation center where the required expertise is available, or the organization may develop its own innovation center unilaterally or in collaboration with other organizations. A dedicated team working on an innovation outside of routine operational distractions can increase the chances of success.

If the innovation is ready for use, the initial action step is to identify the resources (competencies, people, funding) required to support implementation and whether those resources are available in-house. When considering this topic, leaders must assess whether their team has the skills, time, and passion to effectively lead the implementation. Depending on the conclusions drawn at this point, the succeeding action step could be to do one of the following:

1. Purchase (contract for) capabilities, competencies, or resources
2. Recruit individuals with the necessary expertise to join the organization
3. Enter into a joint venture with a partner (e.g., vendor, payer, another provider) to access the needed capabilities or resources
4. Form a consortium of organizations to pool together the needed resources

If, in this process, a decision is made to seek a partner, then appropriate action steps would include identifying criteria to be applied in assessing potential partners, establishing a list of entities to be considered, and objectively selecting the entity that is the best fit.

To implement a clinical or technological strategy, the organization may need to build payer support for reimbursement for that innovation. For example, it may be necessary to build a case that demonstrates to commercial payers that telehealth consultations will reduce costs and improve quality through more rapid diagnosis, prevention of disease progression, avoidance of hospitalizations, and cost reduction for ambulance transportation.

One additional action step should be included for innovations. Take the opportunity to profile the innovation initiative in communications to internal and external audiences. Innovations are typically exciting and interesting. They may motivate staff and donors and help establish your organization as forward-thinking and innovative.

CONCLUSION

Innovation poses both opportunities and challenges for healthcare organizations. Business model changes to address payer–provider alignment, as well as clinical and technological innovation, must be addressed thoughtfully in a planning process. They certainly require the special attention described in this chapter. If successfully integrated, innovation can strengthen a strategic plan and the organization.

REFERENCES

Harris, J. M., and B. Frazier. 2015. "Volume to Value: Choosing Your Strategy for Value-Based Competition." In *Futurescan 2015: Healthcare Trends and Implications, 2015–2020*, 23–24. Chicago: Society for Healthcare Strategy & Market Development of the American Hospital Association and Health Administration Press.

Nagji, B., and G. Tuff. 2012. "Managing Your Innovation Portfolio." *Harvard Business Review*, May, 5–11.

Porter, M. E., and E. O. Teisberg. 2006. *Redefining Health Care: Creating Value-Based Competition on Results*. Boston: Harvard Business School Press.

CHAPTER 13

Future Challenges for Strategic Planners

> The best way to predict the future is to invent it.
>
> —*Alan Kay*

> The future will soon be a thing of the past.
>
> —*George Carlin*

THE STATE OF THE ART IN HEALTHCARE STRATEGY AND STRATEGIC PLANNING

In a highly provocative article, Michael E. Porter, one of the leading authorities on strategy, and his coauthor Thomas H. Lee, MD (2015, 1681), state: "Until recently, most health care organizations could get by without a real strategy, as most businesses understand that term. They didn't need to worry about how to be different or make painful decisions about what not to do. As long as patients came in the door, they did fine, since fee-for-service contracts covered their costs and a little more."

Success came from operational effectiveness: working hard, embracing best practices, and burnishing reputations that attracted both patients and talent. Typically, "strategy" defaulted to having the scale and market presence to secure good rates and be included in networks.

But if that era is ending, the time has come for healthcare organizations to rethink the meaning of strategy. Strategy is about making the choices necessary to distinguish an organization in the competition to meet customers' needs.

A study conducted by Health Strategies & Solutions, Inc., and the Society for Healthcare Strategy & Market Development (SHSMD) in 2005–2006 (Zuckerman 2007) reports that planners and executives believe that healthcare strategic planning practices are effective and provide the appropriate focus and direction for their organizations. Fundamental strategic planning practices appear to be sound, with strategic planning well accepted, used regularly, and integrated increasingly well with other management functions (see exhibit 13.1).

Exhibit 13.1: Evolution of Healthcare Strategic Planning

Dynamic Strategic Management

Stage 4

Strategic Management

Stage 3

- Current average state of the field
- Where is your organization?
- Where should it be?

Mastery of Strategic Planning Fundamentals

Stage 2

Initial Deployment of Strategic Planning

Stage 1

Effectiveness

Best Practices/Advanced Approaches

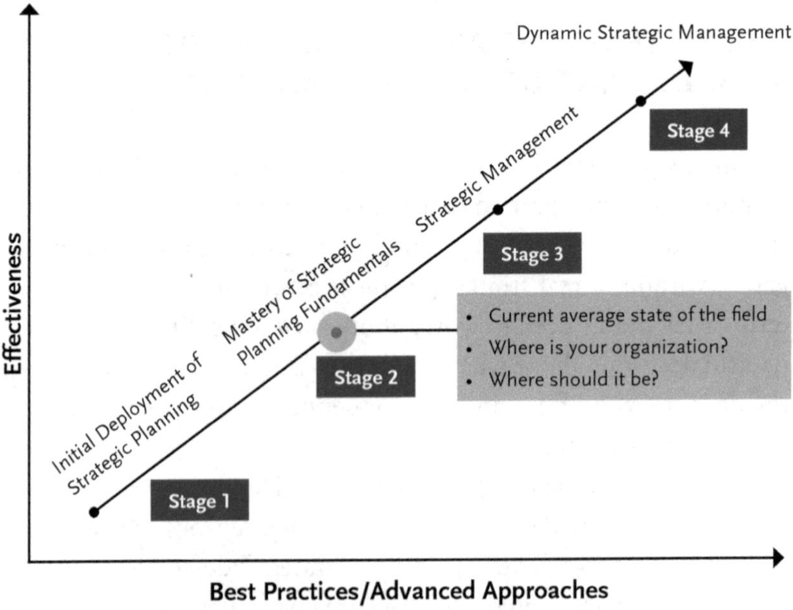

© 2017 Veralon Partners Inc.

But when compared to strategic planning practices outside of the healthcare field, it is clear that healthcare strategic planning has not advanced to sophisticated levels and is far behind what are considered state-of-the-art practices. In fact, the areas in which healthcare organizations seem to do best, according to the survey results—development of mission statements and goals and participation of senior management in the planning process—are rudimentary in strategic planning outside of the healthcare field. Organizations exhibiting more advanced strategic planning would merely think of these areas as the basics, not best practices or even strengths.

Companies that demonstrate pathbreaking strategic planning practices outside of healthcare already embody what are considered bleeding-edge strategic planning approaches among healthcare organizations today, such as attacking critical issues, developing clear strategies, achieving real benefits, and managing implementation.

More important, outside of healthcare, pathbreaking planning practices are characterized by the following five qualities:

1. *Systematic, ongoing internal and external data gathering leads to the use of knowledge management practices.* Rather than the ad hoc data assembly and analysis frequently observed in healthcare organizations, pathbreaking companies outside of healthcare have highly structured systems for continuously gathering information that drives strategic planning. Data gathered are of a breadth and depth rarely seen among healthcare organizations. Once data are gathered, nonlinear analysis is conducted using sophisticated modeling, game theory, and other advanced approaches that far exceed the linear techniques and correlations used in healthcare organizations. The most advanced companies take these efforts to even higher levels by using knowledge management systems that sort information into databases and allow easy access and use by personnel at all levels throughout the organization. Data collection and analysis focus on the market and

external factors and forces, so that decision making is largely driven from the outside, as opposed to the inwardly focused approach more common in healthcare organizations.

2. *Innovation and creativity are prized.* Pathbreaking companies demonstrate the high value they place on innovation and creativity by building a work environment that is receptive to new ideas and looks at alternatives, especially when they create new products and market space. Risk-averse healthcare organizations understand the concepts of innovation and creativity, but putting them into action is another matter. The key issue here is less one of what to do, and more of how to do it. Demonstrating leadership instead of followership and becoming risk tolerant are important first steps for healthcare organizations. Developing a culture that supports, or better yet, encourages risk taking is a necessary prerequisite to progress.

3. *Strategic planning is more bottom-up than top-down.* Leading firms outside of healthcare use a planning process that is increasingly focused in the business units or subsidiaries, with corporate leadership providing high-level direction. This approach allows strategic planning to be more broadly based, meaningful, and substantial, with the real action of planning taking place closer to the customer. Organizational support for initiatives is nurtured when planning has a bottom-up orientation, and implementation may be more successful when planning has been vigorous at lower levels of the organization. Healthcare strategic planning is still too often a top-down process that engenders insufficient participation, awareness, or support from the majority of employees. As health systems consolidate into ever larger entities, there is a risk of even greater top-down planning.

4. *Evolving, flexible, and continuously improving strategic planning processes help organizations adapt more readily.* Pathbreaking companies embrace the inevitability of change and use planning processes with an external orientation. They use external forces and factors to create a platform for change that keeps planning responsive and vital. They regularly revise and upgrade their planning processes and techniques based on their own experiences, observations of other leading companies, and academic research. Many healthcare organizations are content to use the tried-and-true strategic planning processes that worked well historically. Most healthcare professionals are not content with yesterday's operations management and financial planning approaches, so why shouldn't they support similar levels of change in their strategic planning processes?

5. *Dynamic strategic planning has replaced static planning.* Many companies in rapidly changing industries recognize that strategic planning must be dynamic—vision statements must inspire and stretch the organization, goals may need to be revolutionary, strategic thinking is encouraged, decision making is driven down to all levels, and strategic planning is embedded throughout the culture. Strategic planning becomes everyone's job, every day, not just an annual or periodic exercise by executive leaders.

Healthcare leaders must look beyond their own backyards to learn how other highly competitive sectors are spurring organizations to greater levels of growth and success with more rigorous and sophisticated planning. The five qualities discussed here, even when executed at rather basic levels, will go a long way toward helping healthcare organizations experience the benefits that pathbreaking companies realize from their planning processes.

Exhibit 13.2: The Old Guard Versus the New Breed

The Old Guard	The New Breed
Strategic planners' traditional functions, according to a Business International survey, were well defined:	*It can be a struggle for organizations to keep up with an increasingly complex business world. The role of strategic planners should therefore evolve within the framework of traditional functions and be updated with new functions designed to teach organizations to transform themselves:*
Information functions:	**Information functions:**
• Compile information for top managers.	• Compile information for all strategy-oriented teams.
• Research competitors.	• Research competitors and best-in-class benchmarks, including noncompetitors.
• Prepare forecasts.	• Prepare forecasts, especially on internal changes in culture and management style and their effects on environment and performance.
Facilitation functions:	**Facilitation functions:**
• Consult with divisions on how to prepare plans and strategies.	• Consult with divisions on how to improve performance through education, innovation, process management, and total quality management.
• Standardize reporting formats and create common terms of reference.	• Help divisions measure cost of quality, management effectiveness, and team progress.
• Help senior managers convey corporate culture by working cultural factors into the planning process.	• Help senior managers implement changes in corporate culture and measure the impact on performance.
• Communicate corporate objectives.	**Process management functions:**
• Organize and lead planning teams.	• Manage the expansion of the planning process and encourage intelligent employee participation.
Process management functions:	• Develop a process-management methodology and oversee its application to all business processes.
• Manage the planning process.	**Transformation functions:**
• Develop new planning methods.	• Add an internal element (one that asks how to improve as well as what to focus on) to the traditional, externally focused strategic plan. The plan should identify needs and set goals in areas such as management development, benchmarking, process improvement, culture change, and employee participation.
	• Push for recognition that the annual planning cycle is too long, and forecasts too weak, to permit pursuit of a single strategy. Build mechanisms for reassessment into the strategic plan and the organization as a whole.
	• Develop new ways to measure organizational capabilities and performance, focusing on sources of strategic advantage, such as organizational learning rate.

THE NEW STRATEGIC PLANNER

These new perspectives about healthcare strategic planning argue for careful reconsideration of this role in guiding and shaping the strategic planning process. Challenges to the role of the strategic planner have been raised for more than two decades. Alexander Hiam (1993) (see exhibit 13.2) identifies ten principal functions of planners that fall into three basic categories: information functions, facilitation functions, and process management functions. However, these functions do not meet the needs of organizations in turbulent times.

Hiam believes that planners need to take on a new role in which they welcome the input of others, work to convert people to their cause, and shatter received assumptions. They should fulfill the rolls of both active participant and leader in their organizations' transformation.

Henry Mintzberg (1994) argues similarly that the new role of strategic planners—sometimes referred to simply as *strategists*—consists of three elements:

1. *Planners as strategy finders.* Planners need to be active searchers for key strategies that emerge in top management, often unintentionally or that even go unnoticed. Planners need to be constantly on the prowl to discover these strategies "amid the ruin of failed experiments, seemingly random activities, and messy learning" (Mintzberg 1994, 112). Planners should be alert to activities both inside and outside their organizations that can lead to new, important strategies.
2. *Planners as analysts.* Planners have traditionally performed this role of analysis and are quite comfortable with it. However, Mintzberg suggests that planners need to have a broader view of their role in analytical support to offer new models, conceptual approaches, and new processes to address problems.

3. *Planners as catalysts.* Similar to Hiam's recommendations that planners assume a transformational role, Mintzberg (1994, 113) believes that planners need to "encourage managers to think about the future in creative ways." Such planners see their job as getting others to question conventional wisdom and especially helping people out of conceptual ruts.

As we consider where the healthcare field is in terms of strategy development and strategic planning, as well as considering where it needs to go, the results of a survey about strategy practices outside of healthcare may be enlightening. Authors Chris Bradley, Martin Hirt, and Sven Smit (2011) believe that good strategy has ten fundamental qualities:

1. Will your strategy beat the market?
2. Does your strategy tap into a true source of advantage?
3. Is your strategy granular about where to compete?
4. Does your strategy put you ahead of trends?
5. Does your strategy rest on privileged insights?
6. Does your strategy embrace uncertainty?
7. Does your strategy balance commitment and flexibility?
8. Is your strategy contaminated by bias?
9. Is there conviction to act on your strategy?
10. Have you translated your strategy into an action plan?

In an international survey of more than 2,000 executives, the scholars found that nearly two-thirds believed their company's strategy passed three or fewer of these tests, with only about 10 percent saying they passed seven to ten. Given healthcare organizations' relative lack of sophistication in strategic planning, it is likely that they perform even worse. In more recent work focused specifically on healthcare, SHSMD (2014) completed a major examination of the future role of the healthcare strategic planner. The study seeks to answer the question, "Given the evolving changes in the healthcare environment and our desire to enhance the value we bring to the enterprise, how might we, as strategy professionals, reimagine our work?" In summary, SHSMD recommended five areas of future emphasis for healthcare strategic planners:

1. *Be nimble to exceed the rate of change.* Evolve as quickly as the external environment does. Frame problems, ask provocative questions, and move the organization to action.
2. *Tell stories. Create experiences.* Understand needs and motivations in order to compel storytelling. Intentionally design experiences to influence consumer behavior.
3. *Integrate and cocreate.* Facilitate conversations in multilayered and complex organizations, create coalitions, and seek out a diversity of perspectives.
4. *Erase the boundaries of business.* Help develop accessible, integrated systems of care assembled through creative means, such as partnerships and technology.
5. *Generate data-driven insight.* Identify the best tools for collecting, interpreting, and communicating information to deliver insights and better decisions with data.

Looking further ahead and drawing on the more advanced state of strategy development and strategic planning outside of healthcare, Martin Reeves, Knut Haanaes, and Janmejaya Sinha (2015) call for leaders to resist the natural tendency of organizations to hold fast to familiar or historically successful strategies. Instead, readers should encourage a focus on an external perspective, challenging internal biases. Further, with the multiple complex environments of today's markets, leaders need to be the animators of a dynamic combination of multiple approaches to strategy. To carry this out effectively, leaders need to wear eight different hats.

1. *Diagnostician.* Continuously take an external perspective to diagnose the degree of predictability, malleability, and

harshness of each business environment and match this with the required strategic approach for each part of the firm.

2. *Segmenter.* Structure the firm to match the strategic approach to the environment at the right level of granularity, balancing the trade-off between precision and complexity.

3. *Disrupter.* Review the diagnosis and segmentation on an ongoing basis, in line with shifts in the environment, to protect the organization from becoming rigid and to modulate or change approaches when necessary.

4. *Team coach.* Select the right people for the job of managing each element in the collage according to their capabilities and help develop their understanding of the strategy palette, both intellectually and experientially.

5. *Salesperson.* Advocate and communicate the strategic choices as a whole in a clear and coherent narrative to investors and employees.

6. *Inquisitor.* Set and retune the correct context for each particular strategic approach by asking probing questions—not dictating answers—to help stimulate the critical thinking flow that is appropriate to and characteristic of each approach.

7. *Antenna.* Look outward continuously and selectively amplify important signals to ensure that each unit stays in tune with the changing external environment.

8. *Accelerator.* Put weight behind select critical initiatives to speed up or bolster their implementation, especially when the required approach has changed, is unfamiliar, or is likely to be resisted.

Reeves, Haanaes, and Sinha also suggest some tips and traps (see exhibit 13.3) for carrying out the new strategic roles.

Healthcare leaders can find inspiration in the more sophisticated strategic planning approaches of more competitive, market-driven

Exhibit 13.3: Tips and Traps: Key Contributors to Success and Failure for Leaders in Navigating Diverse and Changing Strategic Environments

Tips	Traps
• *Embrace contradictions.* The demands of the many approaches you lead may be diametrically opposed, and that's okay—but tailoring your messages to each environment is critical. • *Embrace complexity.* Introduce complexity in your organization where this will improve the match between environment and strategy without incurring excessive coordination costs. • *Explain simply.* The resulting strategic collage may be confusing to workers and investors; find the common thread to communicate a clear story. • *Look outward.* Use your unique position to counteract the self-reinforcing tendencies of your organization to perpetuate dominant beliefs by keeping the organization externally focused and fluid. • *When in doubt, disrupt.* Organizations naturally become entrenched in their established ways of doing things. In a dynamic world, an overemphasis on continuity is a larger danger than unnecessary disruption.	• *Single-color palette.* Any large organization is probably too complex for a single, unchallenged, and unchanging view of strategy. Avoid oversimplification and uniformity. • *Managing instead of leading.* Getting too deeply involved in managing each approach can prevent you from shaping the strategy collage at a higher level, as encapsulated in the eight roles of leaders. • *Planning the unplannable.* In a world that changes quickly and unpredictably, overinvesting in precise predictions and plans can backfire. An effective leader recognizes that sometimes plans are not the sign of good leadership. • *Rigidity.* Some leaders select an approach but are unwilling to change as new information arises, even though the original course will likely not survive the tides of change.

Source: Reprinted from Reeves, Haanaes, and Sinha (2015).

fields. The qualities discussed earlier, even when executed at rather basic levels, will go a long way toward helping healthcare organizations experience the benefits that pathbreaking companies realize from their planning processes.

CONCLUSION

The good old days of the relatively calm and stable healthcare environment are long gone. Intuition and educated guesses are no longer viable substitutes for sound planning methods. Change is occurring so rapidly that it is impossible to fully understand its scope and impact. With organizations no longer able to rely on the accuracy of long-range forecasts, they must improve their ability to respond to unanticipated changes in the market.

The question is how will change be experienced? According to Gary Hamel and C. K. Prahalad (1994), organizations have two choices: change that happens belatedly, in a crisis atmosphere, or change that happens with foresight, in a calm and considered manner. Will your transformation be spasmodic and brutal or continuous and peaceful?

To quote George Bernard Shaw, "To be in hell is to drift, to be in heaven is to steer." Strategic planning is the vehicle that enables healthcare organizations to steer and have control over their futures. Yet strategic planning is a journey without a specific destination. It will take soul-searching, courage, and commitment to face a future full of uncertainty and potential threats. Strategic planning can help an organization create the road map to guide it through the unknown, balancing the need for articulated and compelling vision and direction with the flexibility to adapt and respond as healthcare is transformed in the coming years.

The effective strategic planner of the future is more than an information gatherer or a guardian of the planning process. She is a leader in management and organizational transformation; a multi-dimensional catalyst of organizational change; and a strategy finder, enabler, and leader. This transformational agenda is ambitious for many healthcare strategic planners, but carries huge potential for personal and professional growth and success.

REFERENCES

Bradley, C., M. Hirt, and S. Smit. 2011. "Have You Tested Your Strategy Lately?" *McKinsey Quarterly*, January, 40–53.

Hamel, G., and C. K. Prahalad. 1994. "Competing for the Future." *Harvard Business Review*, July–August, 122–28.

Hiam, A. 1993. "Strategic Planning Unbound." *Journal of Business Strategy* 14 (2): 46–52.

Mintzberg, H. 1994. "The Fall and Rise of Strategic Planning." *Harvard Business Review*, January–February, 107–13.

Porter, M. E., and T. H. Lee. 2015. "Why Strategy Matters Now." *New England Journal of Medicine* 372 (18): 1681–84.

Reeves, M., K. Haanaes, and J. Sinha. 2015. *Your Strategy Needs a Strategy: How to Choose and Execute the Right Approach*. Boston: Harvard Business Review Press.

Society for Healthcare Strategy & Market Development of the American Hospital Association (SHSMD). 2014. *Bridging Worlds: The Future Role of the Healthcare Strategist*. www.shsmd.org/resources/files/bridgingworlds.pdf.

Zuckerman, A. M. 2007. *Raising the Bar: Best Practices for Healthcare Strategic Planning*. Chicago: Society for Healthcare Strategy & Market Development, American Hospital Association.

Index

Note: Italicized page locators refer to figures or tables in exhibits.

Annual strategic plan review and update (*continued*)

  effectiveness, 224; Jefferson Health (Philadelphia), 219–20, *221*; organizational direction, 218; organizing and setting expectations, 211, 213–14; outcomes for, 209–10; perspective on role of, 224–25; preliminary assessment, 210–11, *212*; process options for, 214–16; strategy formulation component of, 218; time line for, 209

Anthem: strategy statement of, *153*

Ascension Health (St. Louis, MO): Integrated Strategic, Operational, and Financial Plan (ISOFP) for, 220–22; strategy statement of, *153*

Bain & Company, 137

Balanced Scorecard Collaborative, 229

Balanced scorecards, 239, 242, 244–47, 251; business planning component of, *246*, 246–47; communication and linking component of, 246, *246*; defined, 239; description of, 242; development and implementation process, 244, *245*, 246–47; feedback and learning and, *246*, 247; financial measurements complemented by, 242; implementation of, 244, *245*; integrated, iterative strategic management system and, 247; managing performance and effective use of, *246*; strategic management and, 249; translating the vision and, *243*, 244, *246*; use in strategy implementation, 244; use in US companies, percentage of, 242

Balance sheets, management of, *3*, 33–34

Banner Health (Phoenix, AZ): mission statement of, 142, *142*; strategic plan of, 148–49; strategy statement of, *153*; 20-year organizational vision, *149*; values statement of, *145*; vision statement of, *148*

Barrett, Colleen C., 183

Barrows, Edward A., Jr., 137

Bart, Christopher K., 137

Beckham, J. Daniel, 4

Beinhocker, Eric, 89

Bellenfant, William, 172

Benchmarks: comparison to, external assessments and, 119–20

Benefits, of strategic planning, 3, 13–15, 25–45; community benefits, 40–41, *42*, 43–44; financial benefits, 31, *32*, 33–35; identification of benefits, 26–44; operational benefits, 35–36, *37*, 38–40; overview, 25–26; product and market improvement, 27, *28*, 29, *30*, 31; understanding, 13–15, 45

Best practices, in strategic planning, 279, *280*, 281

Big-box stores: clinics in, 261

Birshan, Michael, 91

Bleeding-edge strategic planning approaches, 281

Blue ocean strategy, 94–96; red ocean strategy vs., 95, *96*; value innovation as cornerstone of, 94, *95*

Board, roles in strategic planning, 53–54, 187, 192–98; adoption of strategic plan, 197–98; formal/ informal work sessions with, 196–97; mission statement development, 141, 142, 143; obtain resolution by strategic planning committee, 193, 196; prepare

Clinical and technological innovation, 253, 255, 265–76; addressing in strategic planning process, 271–76; changing nature of, 265–66; environmental assessment: external, 272–73; environmental assessment: internal, 273; impact on access to, and forms of wellness, 254; implementation planning and, 275–76; organizational direction and, 274; physician kiosks, 271; remote monitoring devices, 270; strategic impacts of, 267; strategy formulation and, 274–75; three-dimensional printing, 269–70; types of, 267, 268–69

Clinical integration: alignment concerns and, 176

Clinically integrated networks (CIN), 260, 261, 263, 264

Clinical treatment: clinical and technological innovation and, 267, 268

CMS. See Centers for Medicare & Medicaid Services

Coalition building: strategic planners and, 287

Cognitive function: within organizational vision, 136

Coile, Russ, Jr., 136

Communication: annual update and, 213; balanced scorecards and, 244, 246, 246; in strategic planning, 183; strategic plan rollout and, 199–202, 201; successful plan execution and, 234, 235–36; among team members, 67

Communications plan: potential ideas to incorporate into, 201

Community benefits, of strategic planning, 40–41, 42, 43–44; ambulatory care improvement, 44;

community health improvement, 41, 42; community partnerships, 41, 42, 43; population health management, 42, 43; provision of needed services, 41, 42

Community health, improvement of, 41, 42

Community Health Systems (Brentwood, TN): strategy statement of, 153

Community hospital: organizational assessment of, 2017, 115

Companies: pathbreaking, 281–83. See also specific companies

Competition: based on value, innovation in strategic planning and, 256; blue ocean strategy response to, 94–95; disappearing barriers to, 255; increase in, 18, 19; proactive monitoring of new developments and, 268

Competitive advantages, 5, 122

Competitive disadvantages, 122

Competitors: data sources of, 109, 119; environmental analysis of, 118–19; rigorous analysis of, three-part example from strategic plan, 120, 121, 122

Concluding retreat, 71–72

Consensus: failure of, 12; in strategic planning, 174

Consultants: strategic planning process and, 65

Consumerism: rise of, innovation in strategic planning and, 255–56

Consumer-oriented services design: emergence of, 36

Content ("either/or") thinking: expanded range of, 98–99

Context: annual update and, 213–14

Contingency planning/plans, 91, 171–72; example of, 172, 173; implementation of strategic

"Either/or" thinking, 99

Electronic health records: internal environmental assessments and, 262

Emotional function: within organizational vision, 136

Endowments, 33

Energy: loss of, inconsistent implementation and, 230

Environmental assessments, 105–11; annual review and update and, 216–18; assumptions about the future, 123–27, 129, *129*; creative data gathering for: competitor intelligence, *109*; data requirements for, 107–8, *108*; developing plan for, *106*; external, 116–20, 261, 272–73; future focus of, 123–27, 129; goal of, 7; historical data and, 58; identification of critical planning issues, 129–30, 132; internal, 120, 122, 261–63, 273; organizing data collection process for, 108, 110; poor planning and execution of, 107; primary outputs of, 7; processes in, 107; purposes of, 105; questions examined by, 107; recognizing implications of market change and, 253; in strategic planning approach, *8*

Evashwick, Connie, 6

Evashwick, W. T., 6

"Executing Your Strategic Plan" (Zuckerman), 233

Execution failure: common and detrimental, 13; watching out for signs of, 235

Execution leaders: choosing wisely, 234

Executive champions: strategic goals and, 188

Executive content thinking: categorizing, 98–99

Executive summaries: components of, 193; distribution of, 193; examples of, 193, *194, 195*; integration into strategic plans, 192; length of, 192; overlooking need for, 192–93; stand-alone documents, 192; submission of, 170

Expectations: organizing and setting, annual update and, 211, 213–14

External assessments: end product of, 115–16; environmental, 261; four components in, 116–19; outputs produced by, 120, 122

External interview topics, *111*

External surveys, 73

Facilitation, in strategic planning: identification of facilitators for, 55–56; successful strategic planning process and, 64–67

Facilitators: job description, *66*; three types of skills for, 65

Fads, 255; innovation and, 254; market shifts vs., 253

Failures: identifying, 57

Feedback and learning: balanced scorecard and, *246,* 247

Fee-for-service system: as revenue source, 16

Fee-for-value, 266

Ferris, Nancy, 6

Financial analysis, 172, 174

Financial benefits, of strategic planning, 31–35, *32*; balance sheet improvement, 34; case example of, 34–35; non–operating income improvement, 33; operating margin improvement, 31, 33; use of capital, 33–34; value, 34

Financial measurements: balanced scorecards and complementing of, 242; translating vision and strategy and, *243*

Financial performance: balanced scorecards and, 242; innovation and, 256

Financial planning: balanced scorecard assessment of, 242; independent from strategic planning, 12; integration with strategic plan updates, 249

Financial reserves: business model innovation and, 264

Focus: of effective strategy, 5; loss of, inconsistent implementation and, 230; or niching strategy, 151, 152

Focus Groups: A Practical Guide for Applied Research (Krueger and Casey), 73

Focus groups: strategic planning process and, 73

Fogg, C. Davis, 13, 52, 55, 65, 67, 68, 199, 201, 217, 236, 239

Food and Drug Administration, 266

Ford: vision statement of, *148*

Forecasts: environmental assessments and, 123–26; of healthcare delivery, 116; review of population characteristics, 116

Friedman, Bernard, 151

Fundraising programs, 33

Future: alternative scenarios of, 126–27; assumptions about, 123–27, 129

Future orientation: innovation and, 256; reinforcing, 61

Futurescan: Healthcare Trends and Implications, 217

Game theory, 94

Garratt, Bob, 84

General Electric (GE): mission statement of, 142, *142*

General Motors (GM), 126

Geographic isolation: decline of, innovation in strategic planning and, 256

Ginter, Peter M., 5, 86, 136, 183

Goals, 174, 281; achievement of, 209; annual review and relevance of, 209; business model innovation and, 264; critical issues and, 165, *166–67,* 167, *168*; detailed year 1 implementation plan for new strategic plan and, 185; framework of, 165; identification of, 158–59, 165, *166–67,* 167–70; manageable components of, 171; moving from vision to, 157–59; prioritization process for, 168–69, *170*; setting, basic paths for transitioning to, 162

Goldman, Ellen F., 100

Good Strategy, Bad Strategy (Rumelt), 5

Google: mission statement of, 142, *142*; vision statement of, *148*

Griffith, John R., 242

Haanaes, Knut, 287, 288

Hamel, Gary, 88, 89, 90, 125, 126, 152, 290

Hanford, P., 84; Tools for Thinking Strategically (TTS), 96–100, *97*

Hard data: environmental assessment: competitor intelligence, *109*

Healthcare: investment in, 266

Healthcare delivery in local/regional market: state of, in external assessment, 116–17

Healthcare market: accelerating pace of change in, 255

Healthcare organizations: balanced scorecards and benefits for, 244; increasing size, diversity, and complexity of, 63–64; integration of annual strategic plan with financial planning in, 224; planning retreats and, 71; poor addressing of innovation and, 255

Healthcare reform, 16

Healthcare strategic planning, 16–21; drawbacks to, 281; ensuring applicability of, 19–21; evolution of, 18–19, *280*; history of, 16, *17*; state of the art in, 279–83

Healthcare system product scope framework: modern, *30*

Health Resources and Services Administration: website of, *109*

Health services utilization: forecasting, 119

Health Strategies & Solutions, Inc., 280

Health systems: business model innovation and, 259, 260; entrepreneurial incubators and, 266

Hemingway, Ernest, 183

Hiam, Alexander, 285, 286

High-deductible health plans: rise of consumerism and, 256

Historical data: assembling of, 58; overanalysis of, 58–59; use in environmental assessment, 58

Historical performance: organizational assessment of, 111, 113; as strategic planning process focus, 58

Holistic thinking, 98

Honda: vision statement of, *148*

Hospital-at-home concept: remote monitoring devices and, 270

Hospital discharge databases, state-specific, *109*

Hospitals: aligning physicians with, 50

Hudak, James, 6

Human capital: as operational benefit, *37*, 38–39

Hunterdon Healthcare System, Fleming, New Jersey: community-focused healthcare at, 43–44

IBM (International Business Machines), 126

Idealist leader type, 99

Implementation: business model innovation and, 265; challenges of, 229–30, 232; creating buy-in for, 189, 192; high failure rate in transition from planning, 230, 232; relationship with strategy, *187*

Implementation leader, 233

Implementation planning, 8–9. *See also* Transitioning to implementation; action planning and, *185*; annual review of, 219; clinical and technological innovation and, 275–76; communication during, 183, 199–202; detailed planning during, 183–84

Implementation, steps in fostering success of, 233–36; choosing right execution leaders for, 234; communication and, 235–36; driving the plan down into the organization, 235; execution and, 234; formal, celebratory beginning to planning, 234–35; monitoring system and, 236; moving from strategic planning to strategic management, 236; preplanning and, 233–34; team mobilization and, 234; watch out for signs of execution failure, 235

Implementation subcommittees, 235

Inamdar, Noorein, 244

Incentive-based compensation structures: alignment concerns and, 176

Income, non–operating, *32*, 33

Incubators, innovation and, 266

Independent status of organization: clinical and technological innovation and, 267

Mission: business model innovation and, 263; as directional strategy, 136; strategic planning and, 6

Mission statements, 140, 154, 281; characteristics of, 141–42; content of, 141; definition of, 141; developing, caveats for, 137; development of, 141–43; development process, variance in, 142–43; examples of, 141–42, *142*; guidelines for, 138–41; overall strategic direction for hospital, sample summary, *194*; popularity and prevalence of, 137; vision statements vs., 145–46

Mobile banking, 256

Monitoring system: successful plan execution and, 236

Monopoly pricing: decline of geographic isolation and, 256

"More/less" thinking, 99

Morrison, Ellen M., 151

Multientity systems: emergence of, 19

Multiprovider networks, 260

Nadler, D. A., 15

Nagji, Bansi, 257

National Cancer Institute: website of, *109*

National Center for Health Statistics: website of, *109*

Nelson, Matt J., 172

Niche: definition of, for vision statement, 137

Niching (or focus) strategy, 151, 152

Nike: mission statement of, 142, *142*

Non–operating income, *32, 33*

Nordstrom: strategy statement of, *153*

North Carolina: central, select market characteristics in, *117*

Norton, David P., 137, 242, 247

Nurses: strategic planning process and, 76

Objectives, 157, 174; definition of, 171; detailed year 1 implementation plan for new strategic plan and, 185; establishment of, 171; framework of, 165; for implementation plan, 188; for strategic goal year 1 implementation plan, *190–91*; for strategic planning process, 50; strategy formulation and, 161

O Corrbui, Diarmaid, 184

Online scheduling, 256

Operating margin, 31, *32, 33*

Operational benefits, of strategic planning, 35–40; access, *37, 38*; case example, 39–40; human capital, *37,* 38–39; patient satisfaction, 36, *37*; quality, 36, *37, 38*

Operational effectiveness, 19–20; strategy confused with, 150; true competitive differentiation vs., 19

Operational management: strategic management and, 249

Operational thinking: differentiated from strategic thinking, *85*

Operations: disconnect from, implementation failure rate, and, 230

Opportunism, 152

Organizational assessment: approach to, 111, 113; end product of, 113, *114, 115*; summary categories and, 111, *112–13*; SWOT use in, 111

Organizational behavior: values statement and, 144

Organizational development departments, 65

Organizational direction, 135–54; annual update and, 218; business model innovation and, 263; clinical and technological innovation and, 274; critical outputs of, 154; developing the plan for, 138–39, *139*; development

planning process and, 75–76; strategic planning role of, 55, 196; successful plan execution and, 233

Planning horizons: annual review and update, 209; condensation of, 132

Planning process considerations, major, 63–81; bottom-up vs. top-down strategic planning, 77, 80; evolving and improving the process, 80–81; facilitation, 64–67; key stakeholder involvement, 74–77; overview, 63–64; planning retreats, 69–72; research approaches, 72–74; teamwork, 67–69

Planning retreats: strategic planning process and, 69; types of, 69–72

Planning staff, 65

Population characteristics: in external assessment, 116

Population health management, 259; as community benefit, *42, 43*; shift toward, 27

Portable diagnostic technology, 271

Porter, Michael E., 3, 4, 84, 138, 150, 151, 157, 279

Post-acute care: preferred networks for, 261

Pragmatist leader type, 99

Prahalad, C. K., 88, 125, 126, 290

Predictive analytics: clinical and technological innovation and, 267, *269*

Preliminary assessment: annual review and update, 210–11, *212*

Preplanning: successful plan execution and, 233–34

Preplanning steps, in strategic planning, 49–61; assembly of historical data, 58; avoiding overanalysis of historical data, 58–59; CEO's leadership assertion, 52–53; defining leaders' roles and responsibilities, 53–55; description and communication of planning process, 51; establishment and communication of schedule, 51–52; identification and communication of outcomes, 50; identification of facilitators, 55–56; orientation meetings, 56–57; reinforcement of future orientation, 61; review of past strategy, 57; stimulation of strategic thinking, 59–60

Primary care physicians: internal environmental assessments and, 262

Prioritization: effective, 99; of initiatives, 168–69, *170*

Private equity firms: innovation in healthcare and, 266

Process options for annual update, 214–16; formal and lengthy update process, 215–16; formal but somewhat abbreviated process, 215; informal and very abbreviated process, 214–15

Procter & Gamble: strategy statement of, *153*

Product benefits: of strategic planning, 27, *28*, 29, *30*, 31

Product scope and extent, *28*, 29, *30*

Progress monitoring and review, of strategic plan implementation, 202; during first year, 185–89, *190–91*; frequency of, 202; informal progress reviews, 239; interventions needed for, 239; meeting conduct and, 238; meetings for, 196, 197; ongoing, 236–39; reasons for conducting, 237; rewards and, 239; structured approach to, 238; systems for, 202

strategic planning process and,
76, 77; strategic plan review by,
237; successful plan execution
and, 235–36; updating of strategy
formulation and, 218
Sensitivity analysis: for promotion of
strategic thinking, 91; scenario
planning vs., 92
Service (market) areas, 27, 29
"Seven deadly sins" that doom strat-
egy implementation, 184
Shared savings, 260
Shaw, George Bernard, 253, 290
Shoemaker, Paul J. H., 92, 93, 127
Shortell, Stephen M., 151
SHSMD. See Society for
Healthcare Strategy & Market
Development
Simulation: for promotion of strate-
gic thinking, 91
Sinha, Janmejaya, 287, 288
Situation analysis, 105. See also Envi-
ronmental assessments
Skinner, Wickham, 4
Smart devices: clinical and techno-
logical innovation and, 267, 268
Smartphone-based services, 261
Smartphone technology, 266
Snow, Charles C., 150, 152
Society for Healthcare Strategy
& Market Development
(SHSMD), 280, 286, 287
Soft data: environmental assessment:
competitor intelligence, 109
Sony: vision statement of, 148
Sorkin, Donna L., 6
Souza, Farias, 229
Staff. See also Nurses; Physicians:
alignment issues, 176; leadership,
strategic plan review by, 196
Stakeholder interviews, 110, 111
Stakeholders, involvement in strategic
planning, 11–12, 54, 74–77, 199;

annual review and update and,
209; board members, 74; communication of strategic planning
process to, 51; other clinicians,
76; other management, 76–78;
participation grid, 78; participation in healthcare strategic
planning, 79; physicians, 75–76;
senior management, 76; successful plan execution and, 233, 235,
236
Stanford University: vision statement
of, 148
Static strategic planning: transition
to dynamic strategic planning,
283
"Stay put" thinking, 99
Steele, Richard, 229
Stem cells: three-dimensional printing and, 269
St. Mary's Health: critical planning
issues, 161
Stony Brook Medicine: critical planning issues, 161
Storytelling: strategic planners and,
287
Strategic experimentation, 90
Strategic goals: as directional strategy,
136
Strategic management: annual process components, 250; balanced
scorecards and, 249; benefits
of, 236; relationship to strategic
planning, 236, 247–49, 248;
stages of, 15
Strategic momentum, benefits
of, 15
Strategic plan, financial analysis
example, 181; net financial
impact from major initiatives,
182; strategic financial analysis
projected baseline income statement, 181

Strategic plan, Regional Health System (2017–2022) example, 205–8; factors driving the need for change (2017–2022), 206; introduction, 206; metrics for measuring progress, 208; organizational direction, 207; summary of major initiatives, 208; three broad strategic goals for next five years, 207

Strategic planners: as analysts, 285; areas of future emphasis for, 287; as catalysts, 286; effective, of the future, 290–91; new role for, 283–88, 290; as strategy finders, 285

Strategic planning, 15, 16–21. *See also* Benefits, of strategic planning; Environmental assessments; Implementation planning; Innovation in strategic planning; Organizational direction; Preplanning steps, in strategic planning; Strategy formulation; approach to, *8*; benefits of, 15; best practices in, 279, 281; blue ocean strategy vs., *95–96*; bottom-up vs. top-down, 282; common pitfalls in, understanding, 11–13; contemporary vs. past approaches to, *284*; control over future and, 290; conventional, critique of, 89–90; customized approach to, 21; decentralized vs. centralized, 80; defining, 5–6; description and communication of, 51; dynamic vs. static, 283; ensuring applicability of, 19–21; evolution of, 18–19; history of, 16, *17*; implementation difficulties and, 229–30, 232; independent from financial planning,

12; limitations with, 88; linear vs. nonlinear, 89; meaningful, 59; Mintzberg's critique of, 83–84; primary criticisms of, understanding, 9–11; relationship to strategic management, 236, 247–49, *248*; research approaches to, 72–74; retreat planning component of, 69–72; review of the literature, 136–38; state of the art in, 279–83; steps in, 6–7; strategic formulation phase of, 157–59, *159*; strategic thinking vs., 86–88; surveys, 286–87; teamwork in, 188–89; time frame for, 209; top-down vs. bottom-up, 77, 80

Strategic planning committees, 74; annual strategic plan updating role of, 218; board support for strategic plan and, 197; effective implementation and, 233; goal identification role of, 165; mission statement development role of, 142–43; obtain resolution by, recommending board approval of strategic plan, 193, 196; organizational direction and, 154; oversight role, 54–55; prioritizing of initiatives and, 168–69, *170*; senior management members of, 54–55, 76; strategic planning process and, 67; strategic plan review by, 170, 237; team work by, 188

Strategic plans: adoption of, 170, 197–98; approval of, 186, 197, 198; business model innovation addressed in, 259; critical planning issues common to, 130; develop detailed year 1 implementation plan, 185–89, *190–91*, 202; developing shared understanding about, 64; draft form of, 186, 188, 189, 192–93; duration of, 189, 249; as living documents, 15; monitoring and reporting progress, 186; nonapproval of, 197; progress reports and, 202; review of, 170; rollout of, 186, 199–202; strengthening with innovation, 277; summary, organizational direction, *198*; tactical component of, 169–70; updating, 186, 203; updating, transition to strategic management and, 249

Strategic thinking, 11, 15; advanced, 96–100; benefits of, 15; blue ocean strategy of, 94–96, *95, 96*; contingency planning approach to, 91; decision analysis approach to, 94; definitions of, 83–84; differentiated from operational thinking, *85*; game theory approach to, 94; identifying emerging disruptors and, 91; inserting into management routines of organization, 90–91; matrix of, 87, *87*, 87–88; promoting, 91–100; purposes of, 85, *85*; reinvigorating, 89–90; scenario planning approach to, 92–93; sensitivity analysis approach to, 91; simulation approach to, 91; strategic planning vs., 86–88; tools, 96–100, *97*

Strategy finders: strategic planners as, 285, 291

Strategy formulation, 157–74. *See also* Goals; Objectives; business model innovation and, 263–64; clinical and technological innovation and, 274–75; contingency planning component of, 171–72; critical issues determination

component of, 159–61; execution and, 234; financial analysis component of, 172, 174; forecasting and, 253; goals identification component of, 158–59; moving from vision to goals, 157–59; preparing strategic options and recommendations, 161–63; process of, *160*; relationship to organizational direction, 157, *158*; in strategic planning approach, 7, 8, *8*; updating of, 218

Strategy(ies): defining, 4; development of, 150–52; differentiated from operational effectiveness, 150; effective, key characteristics of, 4–5; execution of, four barriers to, *232*; good, fundamental qualities of, 286; insightful, eliciting, 88–89; kernel of, elements, 5; merger, 262; performance failure of, 230, *231*, 232; relationship with implementation, *187*; rethinking meaning of, 280; revolutionary, 152; translating strategy and: four perspectives, *243*; true, 6

Strategy implementation: "seven deadly sins" and dooming of, 184

Strategy innovation: defined, 89

Strategy statements, 154; examples of, *194, 195*; as executive summary component, 193

Successes: identifying, 57

Success indicator: quantified, for vision statement, 137

Summary categories: possible, *112–13*

Surveys: external, 73; internal, 73; strategic planning process and, 72–73

Sustainability: of effective strategy, 5; strategic planning and, 11

Swayne, Linda E., 6, 86, 136, 183

Value equation, 254

Value innovation: blue ocean strategy and, 94, *95*

Values: competition based on, 256; as directional strategy, 136; financial benefits and, *32, 34*; innovation and, 254, 256; shifting from volume to, 259, 266

Values statements, 140, 154; core of, 144; development of, 143–44; examples of, 144, *145*

Venture capital firms: innovation in healthcare and, 266

Vermeulen, Freek, 83, 90

Videoconferencing: physician kiosks and, 271

Vision: annual review and, 209; balanced scorecard and translation of, 244, *246*; business model innovation and, 263, 264; as directional strategy, 136; impact of innovation on, 274; moving to goals from, 157–59; operational functions of, 136; strategic planning and, 6, 290; translating strategy and: four perspectives, *243*

Vision barrier: strategy execution and, *232*

Vision statements, 154; characteristics of, 146–49; concepts, *147*; developing, caveats for, 137; development of, 145–49; examples of, 137, *148*; mission statements vs., 145–46; overall strategic direction for hospital, sample summary, *194*; popularity and prevalence of, 137; problems with, 146; well-crafted, components of, 137

Visual aids: strategic plan rollout and, 200

Volume: business model innovation and, 264; shifting to value from, 259, 266

Wearables, 266

Welch, Jack, 135

Wells, Denise Lindsey, 248

Yavapai Regional Medical Center (Arizona): Steering Committee scenario exercise, 127, *128*

Zuckerman, Alan, 233

About the Editor and Contributing Authors

John M. Harris, MBA, is a director at Veralon, a healthcare management consulting firm. John has over 30 years of healthcare experience in consulting, management, and entrepreneurship. His work focuses on strategy, mergers and acquisitions, and the transition to value-based payment. He has consulted to health systems and hospitals, accountable care organizations, clinically integrated networks, physician–hospital organizations, and health plans.

Mr. Harris is a faculty member for the American College of Healthcare Executives (ACHE) and regularly conducts seminars on strategic planning and the future of healthcare. He is also a frequent speaker for the American Association of Integrated Healthcare Delivery Systems, the Healthcare Financial Management Association (HFMA), and other organizations, as well as a guest on Sirius Radio. Mr. Harris publishes frequently in *HFM* and has contributed to *Futurescan*.

Mr. Harris has an MBA in healthcare management from the Wharton School of the University of Pennsylvania and a BA from Dartmouth College.

Mark J. Dubow, MSPH, MBA, is a director at Veralon, a healthcare management consulting firm. Mr. Dubow is a national expert in strategy and innovation with more than 30 years of consulting experience in health systems, hospitals, academic medical centers, health plans, post-acute care organizations, and physician organizations.

Mr. Dubow is a frequent speaker for regional and national healthcare organizations. He has taught courses for ACHE since 1999. Over the course of his career, he has published in books and authored more than 30 articles.

Mr. Dubow holds an MBA degree from the University of Michigan, an MSPH, with an emphasis on healthcare planning and policy from UCLA, and a BS in biology from Colgate University.

Carol N. Davis, MSHA, is a principal with Veralon, a healthcare management consulting firm. Carol is an experienced strategy consultant and project director with more than 25 years of experience working with hospitals and health systems, both as a strategy advisor and health system executive. She has led over 250 consulting engagements for community hospitals, health systems, and academic medical centers.

Her work focus includes strategy development and implementation, including affiliations and partnerships, service line and ambulatory care strategy, and clinical integration. Previously, she was vice president of strategic services for a health system in Colorado and has presented at regional and national healthcare conferences.

Ms. Davis holds an MSHA from the University of Colorado at Denver and a BME from the University of Kansas.

Scott Stuecher, MHA, is a manager at Veralon, a healthcare management consulting firm. Mr. Stuecher has over 10 years of healthcare consulting experience and has worked with over 75 organizations across the country, including community health systems, independent hospitals, academic medical centers, and post-acute providers. He manages large, complex strategic and affiliation planning engagements with a focus on helping clients to bridge the gap between analytical conclusions and strategic implications.

Mr. Stuecher has presented at several industry conferences, including ACHE and HFMA. He holds an MHA and a BS in economics from Ohio State University.

Katherine A. Cwiek, MHSA, formerly a manager with Veralon, is senior director of strategic planning and market development at Thomas Jefferson University and Jefferson Health in Philadelphia. At Veralon she consulted to health systems, hospitals, and large physician groups across the country to yield actionable strategy and measurable results. Her current role leverages her planning process expertise and experience in tackling complex issues including clinical program and ambulatory network growth, system integration, physician relationships, and strategic partnerships.

Ms. Cwiek actively publishes in the field and holds an MHSA and a BS from the University of Michigan.